Wellness and Work

Stay Well

Wellness and Work

Employee Assistance Programming in Canada

Rick Csiernik

Editor and Major Contributing Author

Canadian Scholars' Press
Toronto

Wellness and Work: Employee Assistance Programming in Canada
Rick Csiernik, Editor and Major Contributing Author

First published in 2005 by
Canadian Scholars' Press Inc.
180 Bloor Street West, Suite 801
Toronto, Ontario
M5S 2V6

www.cspi.org

Canadian Scholars' Press gratefully acknowledges financial support for our publishing activities from the Government of Canada through the Book Publishing Industry Development Program (BPIDP) and the Government of Ontario through the Ontario Book Publishing Tax Credit Program.

Library and Archives Canada Cataloguing in Publication

Wellness and work: employee assistance programming in Canada / edited by Rick Csiernik.

Includes bibliographical references.

ISBN 1-55130-276-4

1. Industrial hygiene--Canada. 2. Occupational diseases--Canada. 3. Employee assistance programs--Canada. I. Csiernik, Rick

HD7658.W44 2005   363.11'8'0971   C2005-902480-1

Cover design by Zack Taylor, www.zacktaylor.com
Cover photographs, from top to bottom, by David Anderson, Teak Sato, Boris Peterka, Stock.XCHNG, www.sxc.hu
Page design and layout by Brad Horning

05 06 07 08 09   5 4 3 2 1

Printed and bound in Canada by Marquis Book Printing, Inc.

Canadä

For my grandparents Paul and Julia; my great-uncle Tony;
my mother, Violet; and my partner, Debbie:
their work allowed for the creation of this work

Contents

Preface xi

Acknowledgments xiii

INTRODUCTION
1. Wellness and the Workplace
   Rick Csiernik 3

PART I: EVOLUTION
2. The Evolution of Occupational Assistance: From Social Control
   to Health Promotion
   Rick Csiernik 17
3. Disability Management in the Canadian Context
   Tony Fasulo and Sara Martel 45
4. Drug Testing in the Workplace: Issues, Answers, and the
   Canadian Perspective
   Scott Macdonald 57

PART II: STRUCTURE
5. Foundations for Program Development
   Rick Csiernik 73
6. Governance: Best Practices in Policy Development
   Rick Csiernik 83
7. What Are We Doing? The Nature and Structure of Canadian
   Employee Assistance Programming
   Rick Csiernik 101

8. A Review of EAP Evaluation in Canada
   Rick Csiernik 117

PART III: PRACTICE
9. Assessment in an EAP Environment
   Frank MacAulay 133
10. Crisis Intervention in the EAP Context
    Susan Alexander..143
11. Critical Incident Stress Management
    Dermott Hurley, Sandy Ferreira, and Clare Pain 153
12. Brief Counselling in Employee Assistance
    Wayne Skinner...169
13. Brief Treatment for Employees with Low-to-Moderate Alcohol
    Dependence: A Guided Self-Change Approach
    Marilyn Herie..183
14. Intervention in the Workplace
    Penny Lawson 203
15. Depression in the Workplace
    Louise Hartley...209
16. Grief in the Workplace: A Practitioner's Perspective
    Hilda Sabadash..219
17. The Impact of EAP-Based Mediation Services on Employees,
    Families, and the Workplace
    David W. Adams 227

PART IV: CASE STUDIES
18. The Challenge of Rural EAP: The Iron Ore Company of
    Canada
    Debbie Samson...239
19. A Combined Internal/External Model: The St. Joseph's Health
    Centre Employee Counselling Service
    Rick Csiernik, Brenda Atkinson, Rick Cooper,
    Jan Devereux, and Mary Young 245

PART V: CREATING WELLNESS
20. Spirituality and Work
    David W. Adams and Rick Csiernik...257
21. A First Nations' Perspective on Work, the Workplace, and
    Wellness
    Kelly Brownbill 271

22. The Next Step: An Integrated Model of Occupational
    Assistance
    Rick Csiernik 281

List of Contributing Authors..293

Copyright Acknowledgements...301

Preface

Voltaire wrote that work kept us from three great evils: boredom, vice, and need. Philosophers from Marx to Nielsen to Leiss have discussed the importance of work in fulfilling basic human needs and providing meaning to our lives. The importance of work, and its role in resolving needs, is a natural union. However, this endeavour—which meets both our basic and higher-order needs—also may lead us to premature disability and death. The workplace gives us our livelihood, gives us individual and collective meaning, and is a foundation of society; but the high cost of these is that the physical, psychological, social, intellectual, and spiritual well-being of workers may suffer. Historically there has been an underlying acceptance of the risk associated with work, as well as an acceptance that workplace-based incidents will inevitably maim and kill workers. In the twentieth century it became apparent that the risk extended beyond the purely physical dimensions of work to include the psychological and social aspects as well. By the end of the last century one could not discuss work without discussing stress, and the premature disability and death that the stress of work and the workplace environment itself produced. More recently, the ideas of intellectual well-being and the role of spirituality in the workplace have also slowly entered the discourse.

Historically there have also always been groups of individuals who have attempted to mediate the harmful aspects of work. These included members of the labour movement, those involved in self-help, socially minded and orientated corporate leaders, and eventually members of various helping professions. The attempts at assistance have also evolved from meeting only physical needs, to addressing psychological and social needs; the evolution of this assistance now focuses on wellness, combining the traditional dimensions of well-being with intellectual and spiritual health needs.

This enterprise brings together the voices of a range of stakeholders who are actively involved in providing occupational assistance in the workplace, and who share a personal interest in workplace wellness. Their labour provides an understanding of what "wellness" is, along with an examination of the history of occupational assistance in Canada; this ranges from Welfare Capitalism and Occupational Alcoholism to the emerging trends of disability management and drug testing. This collection also provides an insight into how specific workplace-based programs should be structured, and what is actually occurring across Canada, including two specific case studies representing different work sectors from distinct regions of the country. The key practice issues of assessment, crisis work, critical incident stress, formal interventions, and brief therapies are all discussed, along with an examination of depression, bereavement, and mediation. The work concludes with an examination of what could and should be done to create healthier work environments. The conclusion brings us to the next step, an *Integrated Model of Occupational Assistance*. This approach, drawing upon the collective ideas of the previous chapters, illustrates how all workplace stakeholders can join together to create not only well workers and well workplaces, but ultimately well communities.

"Never doubt that a small group of thoughtful citizens can change the world. Indeed, it is the only thing that ever has."

—Margaret Mead

Rick Csiernik
Hamilton, Ontario
October 2004

Acknowledgments

All of the book's contributors wish to acknowledge and thank those persons who are actively endeavouring to bring wellness to their workplaces and to enhance the well-being of their colleagues.

I would also like to personally thank Dr. L. William Lee of the School of Social Work, McMaster University, for his support during my years as an undergraduate social work student; Professor David W. Adams, Professor Emeritus, Department of Psychiatry and Behavioural Neurosciences, Faculty of Health Sciences, McMaster University, and former Executive Director of the Greater Hamilton Employee Assistance Consortium, for the direction he provided me early in my career; and Mr. Abe Friesen, who took a huge risk in hiring me at the Addiction Research Foundation, who introduced me to the world of EAP, and who has always demonstrated true professional style and decorum. I would also like to thank Dr. William S. Rowe, Director of the School of Social Work at the University of South Florida, who has helped keep my academic endeavours moving forward; Dr. John Graham, Murray Fraser Professor of Community Economic Development at the University of Calgary, whose kind words and ongoing support have now spanned two decades; Dr. Susan Silva-Wayne, of Canadian Scholars' Press, for her insights and encouragement; and Ms. Rebecca Conolly, also of Canadian Scholars' Press, for doing all the real work. Without the work and belief of these individuals this work would not have been possible and my own wellness much diminished.

INTRODUCTION

Wellness and the Workplace

Rick Csiernik

Introduction

It is now generally recognized that the workplace exacerbates existing difficulties at the same time as it creates and supports its own unique complement of problems. These problems are caused by the nature of work itself; the necessity to interact at work with colleagues, supervisors, customers, and clients; and the propensity for workers to bring their home life to work and their work life home. The provision of occupational-based assistance is by no means a recent phenomenon. Its roots can be traced to the early 1800s and the emergence and growth of Welfare Capitalism[1] throughout North America. The concept of occupational intervention gained a firmer foothold with the rise of Occupational Alcoholism Programs (OAPs) in the 1940s and 1950s. Policy, procedural, and legislative changes in the United States and Canada in the 1970s opened assistance possibilities to a much wider spectrum of problems, although fixing the maladjusted employee remained the primary focus. What Welfare-Capitalism endeavours and OAPs shared in philosophy and implementation with Employee Assistance Programs (EAPs) was the notion that workers needed to be fixed or molded to some specific conventional form. Minimal attention was paid either to the impact of the work context during this era, or to worker wellness. However, with the move to the "broadbrush" approach and the emergence of Employee and Family Assistance Programs (EFAPs), the focus of workplace intervention has continued to evolve. Environmental factors and situations beyond the worker's immediate control are now being identified as variables contributing to employees' problems (Duxbury & Higgins, 2003; Health Canada, 1996; 1999). In the 1980s and 1990s the beginnings of a health-promotion orientation and wellness programming began to emerge in the workplace, although the primary focus has essentially been only upon physical well-being. The majority of programming has remained focused upon individualizing the problem and seeing the worker as a troubled employee, rather than taking a more ecological approach. Despite some progressive trends, it is still the individual employee who is considered "sick" and who requires reshaping to better fit the needs of the workplace environment. What is now required as we enter the twenty-first century is a more comprehensive understanding of wellness, and of the relationship between wellness and work.

Wellness

The contemporary definition of wellness was premised upon the World Health Organization's (1946: 1) definition of health:

> Health is a state of complete physical, mental and social well-being, and not merely the absence of disease or infirmity.

A complete state of well-being involves wellness of the mind, the body, and the environment; it also involves the integration of family life, community life, and a compatible work interest. Wellness also includes a way of living that maximizes one's potential, helps one adapt to the challenges of the changing environment, and entails a sense of social responsibility (Dunn, 1961). Being "well" constitutes more than merely a state of being not ill, or being "unsick." In fact even prevention alone is an inadequate goal, as prevention can also be viewed as a mostly reactive, defensive response (Ardell, 1977). A wellness approach focuses upon meeting needs in a positive manner and upon pursuing wellness; in this conception the mind, the body, and the spirit are envisioned not only as being integrated, but also as being inseparable. In achieving a state of wellness, individuals need to consolidate not only their physical selves but also their self-image, their work, and their relationships, along with their physical and social environments.

In 1974 a landmark report, *A New Perspective on the Health of Canadians*, was released (Health and Welfare Canada, 1974). This was the first government document to suggest that biological factors along with environmental hazards and lifestyle issues (such as alcohol, tobacco, and other drug misuse and abuse; fitness; recreation; and nutrition) were all determinants both of sickness and of health. The report was also the first to suggest that money should be directed towards a health-promotion strategy, rather than only into traditional health services to serve individuals after they became ill. While the document had minimal initial impact in Canada, it formed the basis for the American Surgeon General's report *Healthy People* (United States Public Health Service, 1979). The focus of that report was a move away from physician-led, hospital-centered treatment to more lifestyle and environmental strategies through which illness could be avoided. This approach has been reaffirmed in a variety of industrialized nations since then, culminating in the World Health Organization-influenced "Ottawa Charter for Health Promotion" (Raeburn & Rootman, 1995).

Wellness is not a static state. Just as there are degrees of illness, so are there also levels of wellness. Positive wellness focuses on the living state rather than on categories of disease that may cause morbidity or mortality. It recognizes that life has extended to the point where its finer differentiation deserves attention (Edlin & Golanty, 1988; Ryan & Travis, 1981). The ultimate goal of behaviour change is to alter the mediating mechanisms of chronic illness, which in turn leads to changes in morbidity, mortality, and longevity. For ultimate success this requires both macro-programming approaches—for example, awareness and education campaigns—and micro-programming approaches—such as focusing on individuals and small groups. Also integral to this process are social network supports, such as those offered by mutual-aid/self-help groups. It is a fact that social relationships further affect wellness by fostering a sense of meaning or coherence, which in turn promotes positive health-related behaviours (Cataldo & Coates, 1986; Hamilton-Smith, 1992; Health and Welfare Canada, 1986).

A holistic and comprehensive concept of wellness, or optimal health, involves an interdependent balance among five areas: physical, emotional, spiritual, intellectual, and social health (see Figure 1.1).[2] Physical health may be thought of in terms of fitness, nutrition, adequate rest and sleep, and medical self-care, including the absence of disease and genetic influences that affect physiological functioning, as well as behaviours that affect biological

Figure 1.1: Wellness

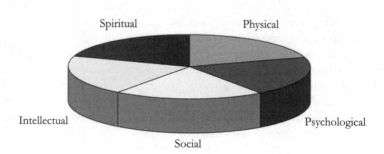

Spiritual   Physical

Intellectual   Psychological

Social

functioning such as smoking and drug use. Emotional or psychological health involves the ability to maintain relative control over emotional states in response to life events, and is associated with stress management and responses to emotional crises. It is the subjective sense of well-being, which includes personality, stress management, life goals, perceptions and feelings, along with health-inducing and illness-preventing behaviours (Green & Shellenberger, 1991). Key characteristics associated with spiritual health include the ability to love, to feel charitable towards and care for others, to feel a sense of purpose, to enjoy inner peace, and to meditate (Adams & Csiernik, 2001; 2003; Sefton et al., 1992). The spiritual dimension of wellness has also been equated with Maslow's concept of self-actualization (Perry & Jessor, 1985). Intellectual health encompasses the realms of education, achievement, role-fulfillment, and career development. It also includes the ability to engage in clear thinking and to think independently and critically (Schafer, 1992). Social health involves social systems that include the following: family, work, school, religious affiliation, social values, customs and social supports, and the ability to interact effectively with others. It entails developing appropriate relationships among friends, families, co-workers, and communities. It also entails role-fulfillment, as well as caring for others and being open to the caring of others.[3]

This holistic view of wellness contrasts with the biomedical model of disease that focuses solely upon biological factors to the exclusion of other practices. When we integrate and maximize social, mental, emotional, spiritual, and physical health, we achieve high-level wellness (Greenberg & Dintiman, 1992). The ideal is to improve all, not merely one or two, at the cost of others. Interestingly, in the workplace co-workers have been identified as being integral to this process as they can contribute to the well-being of each other by providing support and encouragement (Cataldo & Coates, 1986; Schaefer, 1992).

When different components of wellness programming have actually been implemented into North American workplaces, primarily as components of EAPs and EFAPs, the focus has traditionally been on physical health and on changing employee behaviours believed to increase the likelihood and seriousness of illness or other forms of incapacitation at some future point in time. In these instances, wellness criteria are still seen to exist primarily within the person as opposed to within the primary work setting (Ilgen, 1990). However, to create a healthy working environment the end result of work itself should be intellectual, physical, social, emotional, and spiritual well-being. To achieve this end, wellness needs to become incorporated into organizational policies (Herrick, 1981).

Wellness and Work

Historically, the workplace has been a major factor in compromising the health of workers in America. Poor working conditions, long hours, and little regard for the human factor all took their toll on the health status of the workforce. Health and safety improvements were imposed on employers. Business and industry apparently viewed the worker as a static commodity and had little appreciation for the relationship between the health status of employees and productivity and profit.

—James Jenkins, 1988: 125–126

Employers still tend to equate wellness only with physical health, while psychosocial problems are viewed as arising because of the shortcomings of individual employees. However, work itself is inherently stressful. The organization of work also inhibits positive health practices and increases feelings of powerlessness and psychosocial stress (Duxbury & Higgins, 2003; Weinstein, 1986). Among the most predominant workplace stressors are:

i) uncontrollable demands over work (loss of autonomy);
ii) monotonous and repetitive work;
iii) machine pacing of work rhythm;
iv) piece work;
v) the manner in which the workplace is organized;
vi) role conflict/ambiguity;
vii) lack of participation in decision making;
viii) organizational downsizing/reorganization; and,
ix) lack of social contact as part of ongoing work as seen through loneliness and isolation.[4]

In recognition of this, examinations of the relationship between workplace stress and physical and psychological well-being have occurred. Four related sets of variables that influence workplace wellness were found:

i) perceived psychosocial stressors in the workplace and home environments;
ii) personal resources in the form of social support and of self-efficacy as related to work and personal health;
iii) personal health practices including adequate sleep, and use of alcohol, tobacco, and other psychoactive drugs; and,

iv) specific socio-demographic variables such as education and age (Ontario Premier's Council on Health Strategy, 1991; Shehadeh & Shain, 1990).

Stressful life events and excessive demands either at work or outside of it are now commonly believed to suppress one's immune system and lower resistance to infection. While personal susceptibility cannot be overlooked, when demands from personal and work life exceed an individual's ability to cope, or overwhelms his or her existing coping mechanisms, a personalized psychological stress response occurs. This has been associated with increased negative behaviours including the escalation of tobacco and alcohol consumption. Evidence from both human and animal studies have indicated that both personal and environmentally based stress modulate immunity, producing a suppression of the general resistance process and leaving persons susceptible to multiple infectious agents and cancers.[5] Simply, the more negative stress one experiences, the greater the likelihood of the person manifesting a physical illness.

This suppression of the immune system by stress has been linked to a variety of different ailments, including respiratory infections and clinical colds (Cohen, Tyrrell, & Smith, 1991), upper respiratory tract infections, respiratory illness, herpes simplex, and mononucleosis (Jemmott & Locke, 1984), as well as the progression of cancer (Cunningham, 1985). However, as stress reduction is possible at personal, social, and environmental levels, these conditions can all be controlled or minimized. As well, once a person had been diagnosed with cancer, stress-reducing mechanisms can augment traditional medical treatment. Contrarily, social stress, such as isolation or lack of order in one's life, can enhance tumour growth in both acute and chronic forms of cancer.

The way people feel at work is largely a function of conditions at work. Likewise, non-work stress is largely a function of factors that occur outside the job. However, excessive stress in one realm can cross over and interfere with life in the other realm. The stress people experience at work is not simply a reflection of their personal problems, but is accentuated by acute and chronic workplace stressors. Non-work settings typically offer considerably more flexibility and malleability than does the work environment. Work conditions—including a lack of information provision and exchange, unequal power distribution, arbitrary allocation of tasks, role conflicts, poor social relations, physically harsh environments, antagonistic labour–management relations, and lack of job security—are associated with negative physiological changes, somatic complaints, and psychological distress.[6] It becomes obvious that people do not only bring their problems from home to work. Employees also bring work problems home, and the two types of concerns actively interact in both environments.

Karasek and Theorell (1990) studied stress produced by the workplace. They postulated that it is not the nature of work that is the primary risk, but rather the lack of control over how one meets the job's demands and how one uses one's skills. Furthermore, unlike others, Karasek and Theorell argue that it is not necessarily the demands of work, but its organizational structure that is the major culprit in causing stress-related illnesses. A lack of control over work and decision latitude, particularly in instances of high psychological demand, are factors that were found to seriously damage the health of workers. However, it is not senior decision-makers and managers—those normally assumed to be under the highest stress—who suffer the most, but those who have no control over decisions who actually endure the greatest ill health (Table 1.1) (Green, 1988).

The relationship between workplace-induced stressors and an increase in cardiovascular illnesses, including heart attacks and hypertension, has also been empirically demonstrated (Karasek & Theorell, 1990). Job strain may contribute almost as much to the statistical risk of coronary heart disease as conventional risk factors. Ironically, those with the most decision-making responsibility have their stress level increased when given more decision-

Table 1.1 : Factors influencing workers' health by locus of control

EMPLOYER CONTROL

	High	**Low**
High	• work practices • use of protective equipment • workplace hygiene • equipment maintenance and upkeep	• lifestyle • personal health habits

EMPLOYEE CONTROL

Low	• work environment & process • substances used • machinery design • hazard controls • job design	• biological and genetic features • physical and mental impairment • cultural characteristics

Adapted from: Green, 1988.

making responsibility, while those with none have more stress-related illness as a result of being left out of the decision-making process. Thus it appears that both too much and too little control may produce similar threats to wellness.

The relationship between smoking and cancer has been extensively documented and discussed (Blanchard & Tager, 1985; Fielding, 1984). Increased job strain, entailing high psychological demand and low worker control, has also been associated with smoking prevalence and intensity (Green & Johnson, 1990). Thus, any attempts at smoking cessation programs may be undermined if the issue of workplace stress is not also considered. Likewise, modifying employees' job structure in order to increase control and decrease strain can potentially enhance the success of cessation programs. Similarly, reducing stress by fostering a sense of control in a supportive social environment has been shown to assist cancer patients in their recovery (Cunningham, 1985). Social support provided by superiors and co-workers is another ameliorating factor, and has a direct positive impact upon a sense of wellness. Isolated employees face a greater risk of experiencing workplace stress-induced illnesses than those in regular contact with others.[7]

There are three significant components that comprise the psychosocial aspects of the work environment: control, demand, and support. These factors can create a situation of learned helplessness among workers, which can seriously endanger their long-term wellness. A lack of participation in the workplace can also trigger a series of psychoneuroimmunological events that ultimately result in physical pathologies of varying seriousness (Shain, 1992). However, these ideas are not all new as studies dating back to the 1960s explore the relationship between low mental health, psychosomatic symptoms, and the work conditions of automotive workers (Hampden-Turner, 1972). More recently a Canadian study found that workers in four major industries in Quebec had greater rates of distress than the general population. This difference was attributed to workers having too much work and not enough time to complete their tasks, a lack of appreciation for their efforts by colleagues and superiors, inharmonious relations with the employer, inadequate participation in decision making, and limited access to information (Brun, 2002). A positive working environment providing appropriate challenges, which people are actually able to meet, stimulates physical and mental health, while the opposite conditions have negative wellness implications (McCubbin et al., 2003).

Conclusion

It is evident that the workplace is a powerful determinant of all the dimensions of an individual's wellness. The organization of work involves two separate but extremely interactive spheres, the physical environment and the distinct social facet of work (Eakin, 1992). Both need to be considered when analyzing the relationship between wellness and the workplace. The problem of work design is rooted in conventional economic and management theories. This can be traced back to the industrial revolution and Adam Smith's division of labour, but is most obvious in the short-sighted and nearly universal acceptance in North America earlier in this century of Taylorism.[8] The specialization of labour briefly led to higher productivity, but by restricting power and minimizing worker input, thought, and participation, this specialization has sacrificed wellness, and ultimately productivity itself. The structuring of the work environment has led to a virtual global acceptance of the hierarchical pyramid model of administration. Despite being constantly critiqued since their initial postulation, hierarchical bureaucratic structures remain the most prominent industrial organizational model. In comparison to other models, this approach is the simplest to control and historically resembles the feudal control of the peasantry by a lord and his demesne. This model has been called "dysfunctional" and "rigid," as well as incapable of serving the needs of workers; and has been labelled as illness-producing (Karasek & Theorell, 1990; Morgan, 1986). By examining only economic factors and the physical environment of work, conventional theories of production organization have not only adversely affected workers for decades, but also affected industrial productivity throughout North America.

> The lifespan and the health of an individual worker is linked to his or her location in the job hierarchy and to associated factors such as degree of authority, freedom to make decisions and the level of social support in the workplace.
>
> (Ontario Premier's Council on Health Strategy, 1991: 7)

One existing system that has the potential to address the issues surrounding worker wellness and influence processes to enhance workplace wellness is Employee Assistance Programming, but only if it is allowed to evolve beyond its traditional function into an *Integrated Model of Occupational Assistance*.

Endnotes

1. See chapter 2 for a more in-depth discussion of Welfare Capitalism.
2. Sefton, Wankel, Quinney, Webber, Marshall, & Horne, 1992.
3. Green & Shellenberger, 1991; Perry & Jessor, 1985; Schafer, 1992; Sefton et al., 1992.

4. Brun, 2002; Eakin, 1992; Harvey, 1992; Weinstein, 1986.
5. Cohen, Tyrrell, & Smith, 1991; Green & Johnson, 1990; Jemmott & Locke, 1984; Kiecolt-Glaser & Glaser, 1986.
6. Duxbury & Higgings, 2003; Eakin, 1992; Klitzman, House, Israel, & Mero, 1990; McCubbin, Labonte, Sullivan, & Dallaire, 2003.
7. Cohen & Willis, 1985; Johnson & Hall 1988; Marmot & Theorell, 1988.
8. See chapter 2 for a more in-depth discussion of Taylorism.

References

Adams, D.W. & Csiernik, R. (2001). A beginning examination of the spirituality of health care practitioners. In R. Gilbert (ed.), *Health care and spirituality: Listening, assessing, caring.* Amityville: Baywood.

Adams, D.W. & Csiernik, R. (2003). An exploratory study of the spirituality of clergy as compared with healthcare professionals. In G. Cox, R. Bendiksen, & R. Stevenson (eds.), *Making sense of death: Spiritual, pastoral and personal aspects of needs death, dying and bereavement.* Amityville: Baywood.

Ardell, D. (1977). *High level wellness.* Emmasus, Pennsylvania: Rodale Press.

Blanchard, M. & Tager, M. (1985). *Working well: Managing for health and high performance.* New York: Simon and Schuster.

Brun, J.-P. (2002). *The evaluation of mental health at work: An analysis of practices and management of human resources.* Available online at http://www.cgsst.fsa.ulaval.ca.

Cataldo, M. & Coates, T. (1986). *Health and industry.* Toronto: John Wiley and Sons.

Cohen, S. & Wills, T. (1985). Stress, social support and the buffering hypothesis. *Psychological Bulletin* 98, 310–357.

Cohen, S., Tyrell, D., & Smith, A. (1991). Psychological stress and susceptibility to the common cold. *New England Journal of Medicine* 325(9), 606–612.

Cunningham, A. (1985). The influence of mind on cancer. *Canadian Psychologist* 26(1), 13–29.

Dunn, H. (1961). *High level wellness.* Arlington: R.W. Beatty.

Duxbury, L. & Higgins, C. (2003). *Voices of Canadians: Seeking work–life balance.* Hull: Human Resources Development Canada.

Eakin, J. (1992). Psychosocial aspects of workplace health. *Canadian Centre for Occupational Health and Safety.* Newletter. April, 8–10.

Edlin, G. & Golanty, E. (1988). *Health and wellness: A holistic approach.* Boston: Jones and Bartlett.

Fielding, J. (1984). *Corporate health management.* Don Mills: Addison-Wesley.

Green, J. & Shellenberger, R. (1991). *The dynamics of health and wellness: A biopsychosocial approach.* Toronto: Holt, Rienhart, and Winston.

Green, K.L. (1988). Issues of control and responsibility in workers' health. *Health Education Quarterly*, 15(4), 473–486.

Green, K.L. & Johnson, J.V. (1990). The effects of psychosocial work organization on patterns of cigarette smoking among male chemical plant workers. *American Journal of Public Health* 80(11), 1368–1371.

Greenberg, J. & Dintiman, G. (1992). *Exploring health.* Englewood Cliffs: Prentice-Hall.

Hamilton-Smith, E. (1992). Why the word "wellness"? Paper delivered at National Recreation and Wellness Conference, Coburg, Australia, March 12–13.

Hampden-Turner, C. (1972). The factory as an oppressive and non-emancipatory environment. In G. Hunnius, G.D. Garson, & J. Case (eds.), *Workers' control.* New York: Vintage Books.

Harvey, P. (1992). Staff support groups: Are they necessary? *British Journal of Nursing,* 1(5), 256–258.

Health and Welfare Canada. (1974). *A new perspective on the health of Canadians.* Ottawa.

Health and Welfare Canada. (1986). *Achieving health for all: A framework for health promotion.* Ottawa.

Health Canada. (1996). *Towards a common understanding: Clarifying the core concepts of population health—A discussion paper.* Ottawa.

Health Canada. (1999). *Taking action on population health: A position paper for health promotion and program branch staff.* Ottawa.

Herrick, N. (1981). The means and end of work. *Human Relations* 34(7), 611–632.

Jemmott, J. & Locke, S. (1984). Psychosocial factors, immunologic mediation and human susceptibility to infectious diseases: How much do we know? *Psychological Bulletin* 95(1), 78–108.

Jenkins, J. (1988). Health enhancement programs. In G. Gould & M. Smith (eds.), *Social work in the workplace.* New York: Springer.

Johnson, J. & Hall, E. (1988). Job strain, workplace social support, and cardiovascular disease: A cross-sectional study of a random sample of the Swedish working population. *American Journal of Public Health,* 78(10), 1336–1342.

Karasek, R. & Theorell, T. (1990). *Healthy work: Stress, productivity and reconstruction of working life.* New York: Basic Books.

Kiecolt-Glaser, J. & Glaser, R. (1986). Psychological influences on immunity. *Psychosomatics* 27(9), 621–624.

Klitzman, S., House, J., Israel, B., & Mero, R. (1990). Work stress, nonwork stress and health. *Journal of Behavioural Medicine* 13(3), 221–243.

Marmot, M. & Theorell, T. (1988). Social class and cardiovascular disease: The contribution of work. *International Journal of Health Sciences* 18(4), 659–674.

McCubbin, M., Labonte, R., Sullivan, R., & Dallaire, R. (2003). *Mental health is our collective wealth*. Regina: Saskatchewan Population Health and Evaluation Research Unit.

Morgan, G. (1986). *Images of organization*. Beverly Hills: Sage.

Ontario Premier's Council on Health Strategy. (1991). *Nurturing health: A framework on the determinants of health*. Toronto.

Perry, C.L. & Jessor, R. (1985). The concept of health promotion and the prevention of adolescent drug use. *Health Education Quarterly* 12(2), 169–184.

Raeburn, J. & Rootman, I. (1995). *People-centered health promotion: A Guide for students and professionals*. Toronto: Centre for Health Promotion, University of Toronto.

Ryan, R. & Travis, J. (1981). *The wellness workbook*. Berkeley: Ten Speed Press.

Schafer, W. (1992). *Stress management and wellness*. Toronto: Harcourt Brace Jovanovich.

Sefton, J., Wankel, L. Quinney, H., Webber, J., Marshall, J., & Horne, T. (1992). Working towards well-being in Alberta. Paper delivered at *National Recreation and Wellness Conference*, Coburg, Australia, March 12–13, 1992.

Shain, M. (1992). *Labour law is a hazard to your health: Implications for reform. Issues in health promotion series*. University of Toronto: Centre for Health Promotion.

Shehadeh, V. & Shain, M. (1990). *Influences on wellness in the workplace: A multivariate approach*. Ottawa: Health and Welfare Canada.

United States Public Health Service. (1979). *Healthy people: The Surgeon General's report on health promotion and disease prevention*. Washington, DC: Department of Health, Education and Welfare.

Weinstein, M. (1986). Lifestyle, stress and work: Strategies for health promotion. *Health Promotion* 1(3), 363–371.

World Health Organization. (1946). *Constitution*. New York.

Part I

EVOLUTION

2

The Evolution of Occupational Assistance:
From Social Control to Health Promotion

Rick Csiernik

Introduction

Needs manifest themselves in all facets of life. As work outside the home and in the employ of third parties grew in Canada and the United States, so did the realization that the satisfaction of needs would become, in part, the responsibility of employers. The exchange of labour for money allowed individuals to make purchases that met basic needs. However, the workplace also took on a role in resolving problems and meeting a range of personal needs, a role that has evolved continuously since the beginning of the industrial revolution. There has also emerged a historic relationship between occupational assistance and mutual aid/self-help in North America through four distinct eras: Welfare Capitalism, Occupational Alcoholism, Employee Assistance, and workplace health promotion. Each phase in the evolution of occupational assistance has witnessed the interaction of personal, organizational, and societal influences that have provoked and motivated different stakeholders in the workplace to become involved in initiating and developing programs. Among the most prominent and integral players throughout this entire evolutionary process have been self-helpers and mutual-aid groups, although recently their importance and influence have lessened. This review highlights the value of mutual aid/self-help within occupational assistance programming and the reasons why it needs to continue to be a core component in creating a well workplace in the twenty-first century.

Welfare Capitalism

At the onset of the Industrial Revolution, little value was attributed to workers; employees were viewed as being expendable and easily replaceable.

They were part of the industrial machine. However, the expansion of industry in the late 1800s in North America led to an increasing number of immigrants and women entering the paid labour force. This changing face of the workforce was compounded by increases in labour unrest, with nearly 23,000 strikes affecting 117,000 worksites throughout North America between 1880 and 1900 alone. Some employers responded to this by hiring private police forces and by directing violence against striking workers. A vastly different response by other employers was the development of industrial welfare initiatives. Welfare Capitalism was a nineteenth- and early twentieth-century North American employer mechanism whose motive was to obtain worker loyalty by meeting a smattering of the basic needs of employees through programming initiatives; these initiatives were neither a necessity of the industry nor required by law (Brandes, 1976).

In spite of the humanitarian overtones, the underlying motivation of Welface Capitalism was to create a healthy, hard-working, efficient, orderly, productive, and diligent non-unionized workforce that would not question management initiatives, decisions, values, or ideals. Paternalism was an intrinsic element of Welfare Capitalism. Owners viewed their acts as a means to produce a contented and subdued labour force, whose needs would be met and who would therefore have no need to organize itself, or turn to labour unions to assist in fulfilling their needs (Googins & Godfrey, 1987; Popple, 1981; Scheinberg, 1986). Paternalism motivated companies such as the Washington, Idaho, and Montana Railway and the Potlatch Lumber Company to create "dry zones" around their worksites and to create company towns that outlawed taverns and alcohol within the town limits (Petersen, 1987). Paternalism fostered a culture of dependence among workers, while the majority of owners presumed that their employees should have felt privileged to be working for a company or living in a company town that provided so much for them in return "only" for their labour (Allen, 1966). Other owners, especially those with a strong Christian philosophy, believed it was their obligation to exercise control of both the internal and external affairs of their employees, and to create both a higher moral plane and a greater sense of responsibility among workers (Boyer, 1983; McGilly, 1985). Despite the resentment these attempts at social engineering fostered among workers, paternalism and Welfare Capitalism were considered by numerous nineteenth-century businessmen to be a "moral responsibility, protecting society while furthering business" (Garner, 1984: 53). As new immigrants flooded North America, paternalism became the instrument for socializing them into the established cultural norms. It became the mechanism to control and "Americanize" the increasingly immigrant workforce (Allen, 1966).

Predominantly, only basic needs were met through Welfare Capitalism programs, including the establishment of non-profit lunchrooms, shower facilities, and company stores. However, some owners went further and established medical clinics staffed by company nurses and physicians. Other management initiatives extended financial benefits to workers through the provision of pension plans, profit-sharing schemes, sick benefits, and even paid vacations. Some programs moved beyond meeting basic needs by providing recreation facilities, adult education programs, schools for the children of workers, libraries, and welfare secretaries (Googins & Godfrey, 1987; McGilly, 1985).

In 1875 Mrs. Aggie Dunn was hired to look after the needs of the young women working for the H.J. Heinz pickle factory and living in the company dormitory. She became the first welfare secretary in North America, acting as a liaison between the male management and the predominantly female workforce. The primary function of welfare secretaries was to be a socializing and controlling influence on the workforce, with an emphasis placed upon meeting the needs of female and immigrant workers. The welfare-secretary position eventually developed into a role to assist in creating more efficient workers and to maintain good physical health and moral hygiene so that employees could be as productive as possible (Brandes, 1976; Popple, 1981; Thomlison, 1983). While the exact nature of the role of many of these welfare secretaries was undefined, their responsibilities can be placed into four categories of health and welfare provision:

i)   physical: safety, sanitation, and housing;
ii) cultural: recreation, education, and socialization of North American values;
iii) personal: casework-like services for employees and their families; and,
iv) economic: administration of loans, pensions, and related financial benefits (Carter, 1977).

The function of welfare secretaries involved what could be defined as the beginnings of casework practice and rudimentary group work. Many welfare secretaries were encouraged to develop education and social-support groups as a technique for problem resolution; in fact, any activity that minimized the time employees spent in taverns was generally looked upon favourably by employers. Welfare secretaries were the initial internal professional providers of occupational assistance, and by the onset of World War I there were approximately two thousand welfare workers in industry throughout Canada and the United States (Sonnenstuhl & Trice,

1986). While many had no formal training, the major sector of employment for graduates from the New York School of Social Work during this era was industry. In fact, Carter (1977) claimed that the first North American usage of the term social work in the late 1800s was a direct translation of the German phrase "arbeiten sozial," the practice of providing housing, canteens, and health care by German manufacturers to their employees.

The primary focus of mutual-aid groups during this period was economic concerns. The modern concept of self-help had not yet taken root and the types of activities that could be classified as mutual aid were almost exclusively related to financial self-help initiatives, including union organizing and economic co-operatives (Katz & Bender, 1976). In the nineteenth century, "Friendly Societies" emerged to assist the working class in coping with adverse living conditions, and became the most important British voluntary association of the nineteenth century, promoting both thrift and mutual aid. They were attempts by workers to meet their social and convivial needs, as well as to insure against the hazards of sickness and death, as employers offered inconsequential, if any, long-term economic security. The Societies increased in number, size, and prominence as industrialization, and consequent alienation, increased. Friendly Societies did not owe their origins to government, nor to private benevolence, as the plan originated among those it was intended to serve. A key social component was the monthly club nights, with sociability being an important motivating aspect for joining. Friendly Societies became so allied with local pubs and with drinking and celebrating that questions were put to some groups regarding the over-allocation of funds to alcohol (Gosden, 1973). However, by the end of the nineteenth century there was a growing realization that this mutual-assistance effort was not adequately preventing large numbers of injured workers and their families from becoming poverty-stricken (Rimlinger, 1983).

Friendly Societies did not spread throughout North America, though other types of economic self-help initiatives did arise during the 1800s. These included irrigation and farming co-operatives, and the first North American industrial trade union, the Knights of Labour. The foundation of the Knights was also primarily motivated by economic self-help principles (they did, however, establish a formally organized and entrenched leadership hierarchy; this structure would eventually contribute to the collapse of the group). Nevertheless, this early craft and trade union embodied many of the principles of contemporary mutual aid (Katz & Bender, 1976; Romeder, 1990).

One particularly interesting Friendly Society was the Independent Order of Rechabites formed in 1835. By World War II, the Rechabites had a membership of approximately half a million. The motivation behind this group, beyond establishing basic financial security for its membership, was self-protection for those who had joined: the Rechabites were also a temperance movement, and offered sanctuary for those who did not wish to enter or return to the pub life (Gosden, 1973). A similar movement arose in the United States during the same period of time. Founded in 1840, the Washingtonians based their group on a format culled from Christian religious roots. Washingtonians advocated total abstinence from alcoholic beverages, and targeted the workplace as an essential area to spread their message. They actively sought out excessive drinkers from work settings to counsel and aid. The Washingtonians used group meetings to provide support to those attempting to give up drinking and to assist others in maintaining their abstinence. While political and religious disagreements eventually led to the demise of the Washingtonians, a fellowship with similar motives soon followed: the Oxford Group targeted primarily college students and graduates. Included in their temperance message was the idea that people are sinners, but that they could be redeemed through public confession. A fundamental belief of Oxford Group members was that those who were converted must move on to assist others in changing (Garnter & Riessman, 1976; Presnall, 1981; Trice & Schonbrunn, 1988). In an era when neither the economic nor social welfare of workers was a prominent industrial concern, these two groups set the stage for the emergence for what was to become the world's most influential self-help group, one that would not only serve as a template for mutual aid for decades, but also irrevocably shape occupational assistance.

By the turn of the century, the workplace was seen less as the focal point for drinking, and increasingly as a place where everything was done to discourage the use of alcohol. This change was motivated by several factors: the increasing strength of the prohibitionists and the social gospel movement, the importing of workers' compensation legislation initiatives from Europe, the short-lived mental-hygiene movement that engaged mental health practitioners to eliminate eccentricities from persons employed in industry, and the developing field of personnel administration inspired by Taylor's *Principles of Scientific Management* (Googins & Godfrey, 1987; MacKintosh, 1939; Preston & Bierman, 1985; Scheinberg, 1986). In Canada, union-led initiatives, particularly by the Knights of Labour, also acted to discourage excessive drinking by workers. Labour leaders felt inebriated workers were too easily made pawns by the owners of the means of production who would supply cheap liquor instead of adequate wages (Kealey & Palmer, 1982).

An aspect of Welfare Capitalism rarely discussed, which was also associated with temperance ideals, involved the contracting of service providers external to the workplace. The Young Men's Christian Association's (YMCA) growth throughout North America was not happenstance: in the late nineteenth and early twentieth century, the YMCA was commissioned by large businesses, primarily railway interests, to provide welfare services for their workers, given that there were few recreation, social, or housing alternatives for this segment of the workforce. The YMCA developed a distinct Railroad unit to follow the rail workers throughout North America as the train system was expanded. The first railroad YMCA was established in Cleveland in 1872, and by 1879 there were 39 YMCA railroad centres. By the end of World War I the YMCA employed nearly 250 professional industry secretaries supported by over 4,000 volunteers, mostly students from colleges and technical schools, in 154 locales. This arrangement relieved larger multi-centre companies of administrative burdens while also allowing smaller organizations to share in a broad range of welfare programs, including housing of their workforce in a morally correct, sober, Americanizing environment. Religious-education classes were also used to reinforce the idea that good Christians did not strike against their employers (Brandes, 1976; McGilly, 1985). As the YMCA's programming expanded, companies would turn over established facilities to allow this external "independent" agency to administer them (Allen, 1966). Similarly, the Young Women's Christian Association (YWCA) provided shelter for those women who were unable to find work in industrial centres, were pregnant and single, or who had become prostitutes and were attempting to change their lifestyle (Zahavi, 1988). Thus, it can be argued that the YMCA and YWCA were the inaugural external, third-party providers of occupational assistance in North America.

The emergence of the YMCA and YWCA programs was one of several reasons behind the demise of the role of the internal welfare secretary. The increasing availability of both publicly- and privately-funded community-based social services and mutual-aid/self-help associations in large urban areas also allowed employees to seek help from others than those working for their employers to meet their needs. The inclusion of economic welfare responsibilities had already begun to move the duties of welfare secretaries away from social-work-orientated intervention and more towards the emerging discipline of personnel management. Some welfare secretaries were not only responsible for administrative functions including managing employee welfare benefits, lunchroom activities, and medical clinic activities, but were also becoming involved in training staff, job assignments, and even hiring. Henry Ford employed them to evaluate the moral fitness of his employees. Those deemed morally fit and deserving could earn up to $5.00 per day while those falling short of Ford's criteria could earn only a daily maximum of $2.60. Thus, tensions that the welfare secretaries were supposed to defuse between management and labour were often heightened by these tasks, and the position was soon labelled anti-union. With the increasing prominence of Taylorism and Scientific Management principles, the human-welfare component of the position was further eroded (Carter, 1977; Googins & Godfrey, 1987; Shain & Groeneveld, 1980).

Slowly the impetus behind Welfare Capitalism drifted away from procurement and protection of labourers, to being another kind of management tool. Its overriding objectives became to avoid labour disputes that could paralyse an industry and to increase the productivity through the intellectualization of individual workers (Garner, 1984). The motivation became not only to create a stable, loyal, and sober workforce, but also to undermine Bolshevism, Radicalism, Socialism, and all other "isms" that might disrupt the labour community (Petersen, 1987; Zahavi, 1988). Welfare Capitalism, with its paternalistic overtones, tied benefits to allegiance, obedience, and co-operation, and not to sharing, participation, consensus, or any type of discourse. It was during, and partially because of, the depression of the 1930s that this paternalistic era began to decline. With the introduction of the National Labour Relations (Wagner) Act of 1936, part of the American "New Deal," and the Canadian War Labour Order of 1944, there were even fewer returns for employers who still engaged in Welfare Capitalism activities. The energies of owners now became almost exclusively devoted to overtly meeting their own needs rather than attempting to placate workers.

While some of the motivating factors behind Welfare Capitalism were undeniably noble, even verging on altruistic, overall, the movement can be labelled as a largely paternalistic endeavour, which eventually led to the co-option of social workers and other helping professionals involved in the field. It created a coercive, autocratic, and feudal organizational environment, which perpetuated a system of labour–management relations in which the distribution of both powers and rewards was decidedly unequal. Mutual-aid/self-help initiatives sponsored or supported by employers were also primarily used as work socialization mechanisms and as another vehicle to stave off organized labour or co-operative ventures.

Occupational Alcoholism Programming

In 1935, as the last vestiges of Welfare Capitalism were winding down, a historic meeting was taking place in Akron, Ohio. Bob Smith, a physician, was talking with a stockbroker, Bill Wilson. The discussions of these two

white Protestant men would profoundly shape the way alcohol treatment
would be defined and researched, the way in which substance abusers
would be treated, the unfolding of the self-help movement, and the
further development of occupational assistance. On the eve of a major
transformation of the North American workforce came the emergence
of the inaugural contemporary mutual-aid/self-help group, Alcoholics
Anonymous (AA).

The history and growth of occupational assistance is interwoven
with Alcoholics Anonymous. Both Bill Wilson and Dr. Bob Smith had
participated in the Oxford Group prior to their fateful encounter in Ohio.
Their use of core self-help principles—sharing of past experiences, mutual
support, and the helper–helpee philosophy—was fundamental in assisting
them to maintain their sobriety (Gartner & Riessman, 1977; Katz & Bender,
1976; Wilson, 1957). In the spirit of the Washingtonians and Oxford
Group, they were determined to help others experiencing similar problems
with alcohol misuse and abuse. AA was not intended as a rejection of
professional treatment, but rather as an alternative; in reality, however, no
effective treatment of any type existed during this period. The motivation
behind AA was to use collective experience, fellowship, and sociability to
assist those with a common problem to help each other cope with their
situation on a daily basis. To build a sense of mutuality and give some
order, twelve steps and traditions were developed that could be used and
followed by others attempting to maintain their own sobriety (Robinson
& Henry, 1977). Partial responsibility for the growth and development of
occupational assistance programming during this era can be attributed to
the individual motivation of AA members. The twelfth step states:

> Having had a spiritual awakening as the result of these steps, we try to
> carry this message to alcoholics and to practice these principles in all our
> affairs.
>
> Alcoholics Anonymous (1946: 15)

Another significant organizational factor that influenced occupational
assistance programming was the overwhelming emphasis placed by labour
unions on business unionism, particularly in the United States during
the late 1930s. Historically, labour in Canada had a tradition of social
involvement, particularly through its association with the social gospel
movement. One reason Welfare Capitalism had not been as dominant
in Canada as in the United States during the early 1900s was the greater
provision and securement of social benefits by organized labour. However,
the disempowerment of unions began in Canada with the failure of the

1919 Winnipeg General Strike. It was further weakened by the loss of momentum in the social gospel movement, and was nearly fatally disabled by the impact of the 1930s depression (Allen, 1971). In the place of social activism, Gomperism became the dominant theme in the North American union movement. The exclusive mandate under Samuel Gompers, President of the American Federation of Labour during the 1930s, was the acquisition of enhanced financial benefits and working conditions; the "pay packet and lunch pail" philosophy superseded the broader Canadian labour goals of social justice and equality. Gomperism greatly negated labour's role in providing occupational assistance to its membership (Kerans, Dorver, & Williams, 1988; Robin, 1968).

However, with the end of the 1930s and the onset of World War II, management's greatest asset was vastly diminished. No longer was there an overly abundant supply of surplus labour. Those who had been considered unemployable five years earlier were now in great demand. Individuals who had previously been labelled as "marginal" employees were suddenly essential to the wartime workforce. If one recalls the labour influx of the late 1800s inspiring the introduction of Welfare Capitalism, it is no surprise that new problems surfaced with this new wartime labour influx. The most readily identifiable dilemma was the alcohol-dependent employee. Employers were faced with employees who would not show up for work, or who were unable to perform; the problem was worsened by the fact that there were no longer plentiful spare bodies with which to replace them. These outcasts were now needed, if not necessarily wanted, in the workplace (Corneil, 1984; Trice & Sonnenstuhl, 1985).

In 1939, by which time the Akron, Ohio group had grown to approximately 100 members, the Alcoholics Anonymous moniker was formally adopted. Soon afterwards, Bill Wilson himself began to meet with corporate leaders to promote the concept of AA in the workplace. This included the chairman of E.I. du Pont de Nemours and Company, Maurice du Pont Lee. It was du Pont Lee who first hired a member of AA, Dave Meharg, to actually work in the medical department to provide assistance and to refer alcoholic employees for treatment. E.I. du Pont de Nemours was also the first company to enter into a formal agreement granting time off from work for employees who wished to participate in an Alcoholics Anonymous meeting during their shift. Several other large American corporations, including Kodak, Allis-Chalmers, Armco Steel, Consolidated Edison, and Western Electric, whether by accident, as a calculated risk, or as an act of corporate social responsibility, also began to hire recovering alcoholics. These employees, placed either in the personnel or medical departments, "treated" alcoholics in the only method of the era, Alcoholics

Anonymous. Corporate medical directors without staff affiliated with AA also turned to the self-help group because of their general inability to effectively treat employed alcoholics (Dunkin, 1982; Scanlon, 1986; Trice & Sonnenstuhl, 1985).

Employees active in AA not only intervened with other alcoholic employees, but also helped to establish both on-site and external community-based groups, while also attempting to act as role models for those who did not realize or acknowledge their alcohol dependency. As this method of prescribed workplace-based intervention became more widespread, it became formally known as Occupational Alcoholism Programming (OAP). The early years of OAP relied upon individual AA members assisting fellow employees, while organizationally, managers ferreted out those who would not seek help. The driving motivation to provide assistance and meet the needs of troubled employees came not from industry, organized labour, or government, but from recovering alcoholics who wished to share their newfound sobriety with others (Baxter, 1984). The motto became "get alcoholics into treatment while they still have something to lose, something at stake" (Shain, 1978: 2). AA provided worksites with a system for responding to alcohol dependency, a practical method for treating employed alcoholics, and human resources to do so. During the formative years of OAPs, AA supplied the labour power to programs, allowing them to mature and demonstrate their worth (Trice & Sonnenstuhl, 1985). While restorative in nature, AA was, and still is, exclusively treatment-orientated. However, this method of self-help only has utility once an employee's problem has already reached a significant level and is readily discernible. Its exclusionary nature forces it to be concerned only with the treatment of alcohol-dependent individuals, and not with the structural workplace and societal problems that contribute to alcohol misuse and abuse (Katz & Bender, 1976).

Bell Canada, during the 1940s, was the first reported Canadian employer to initiate an OAP. Under the directorship of Dr. Harvey Cruickshank, a psychiatrist, a program was established within the medical department, although with no recognition by, or formal assistance from, AA. The program evolved from a study conducted by Cruickshank on the main causes of illnesses and absences, and their effects upon business. Employees who scored high in both sickness and absenteeism were predominately ones with alcohol-related problems. Subsequently, Bell Canada instituted a policy recognizing alcoholism as a health problem that was treatable and allowed those suffering from the affliction to be eligible for sick benefits and exempt from standard disciplinary procedures during their period of recovery (Lindop, 1975; Trice & Schonbrunn, 1988). A few American organizations followed a similar path in hiring psychiatrists or industrial psychologists to intervene with alcohol-dependent employees. This industrial mental-health counselling movement was short-lived, as the approach was generally ineffective in recognizing alcohol-dependent individuals, and the techniques employed were not productive in assisting those few who were identified (Presnall, 1981).

During the 1940s and 1950s there was little independent initiation of OAPs by Canadian companies other than those who were branch plants of larger American corporations, such as Kodak Canada, Gulf Canada, and Canadian Pittsburg Industries (Caldwell, 1977). It was the Ontario Addiction Research Foundation (ARF; now the Centre for Addiction and Mental Health) which pioneered a wider appreciation for and understanding of this new variation on occupational assistance. During the 1950s, ARF's major occupational program was to link employees with drinking problems with an AA contact. In the 1960s, the first regional consultant to industry and labour was hired to promote Occupational Alcoholism Programming. This initiative was copied ten years later in the United States, and fuelled the emergence of Employee Assistance Programs (EAPs). Hamilton, Ontario was chosen for a pilot project because of its large, diversified manufacturing base. During the 1960s several initiatives were launched to train labour and management in identifying problem drinkers, and establishing referral routes through industrial medical departments. In fall 1973, the Hamilton Community Coordinating Group, which became the EAP Council, was formed to begin a community development project designed to enhance the effectiveness of programs through professional development activities, and to increase the profile of Occupational Assistance Programming (Bennett, 1975; Massey & Csiernik, 1997).

Companies in the vanguard of occupational assistance were moving from "Theory X" of Management towards "Theory Y" (McGregor, 1960). Managers working on a Theory X basis believed that employees were inherently unmotivated, immature, innately lazy, did not wish to work, were resistant to change, and did as little as possible to gain as much as possible. Businesses organized on a Theory X model believed that workers needed direction and wished to avoid responsibility, security being their paramount need. Theory Y took a less extreme, more humanistic position. Its philosophy declared that the expenditure of physical and mental effort in working was as natural as play and rest. One did not need to punish workers to motivate them, as under the proper working conditions all people learned and actually wanted to contribute. Y theorists had a more integrative perspective, postulating that a majority of employees strove towards self-direction and responsibility in their work. The majority of employees wished to be creative and worked to meet not only their own personal goals and needs, but also the goals that were beneficial to the entire workplace. Thus, external control and the threat of punishment were not the only means for bringing about movement towards organizational objectives. Theory X traces its philosophical roots to Taylorism, while Theory Y became the jumping-off point for the more progressive interpretation of industrial development, demonstrated by organizations adopting Total Quality Control initiatives (Corneil, 1984; Haney, 1979; Juran, Gryna, Jr. & Bingham, 1951, McGregor, 1960).

While social work in its infancy had been a foundation for earlier workplace interventions, there was no designated role for the profession during this stage, with some minor exceptions. Bertha Reynolds pioneered direct social-work practice while employed by the National Maritime Union's United Seaman's Services during World War II. Throughout the course of the war, more than 5,000 union members were killed. Along with her staff of six assisted families, Reynolds made claims for losses, injuries, and deaths, and dealt with bereavement, while also attempting to locate sailors lost abroad. Social workers played a similar role for members of the armed forces and their families (Carter, 1977; Masi, 1983; Straussner, 1989; Thomlison, 1983).

With minor exceptions, such as employing Reynolds and her colleagues, labour's contribution to meeting the needs of workers during this phase of occupational assistance development was also minimal. Overall, the North American union movement was still motivated by a Gomperism philosophy. Unions continued to focus their efforts on enhancing basic needs through the collective bargaining process, and were not typically invited by management to assist in developing OAPs, and rarely did organized labour actively lobby to be part of the process. This further allowed the entrenchment of workplace intervention as a role for supervisors and managers, much to the chagrin of segments of the rank and file, as well as more radical labour locals. These groups asserted that OAPs were nothing more than witch hunts to detect and discharge unwanted union members, under the guise of addressing alcohol-related problems (Corneil, 1984).

The move from Welfare Capitalism to Occupational Alcoholism Programming did, however, see a shift in emphasis from exclusively management needs to a greater focus on individual needs. The mood of this period was set by the philosophy of Alcoholics Anonymous. Individuals were attempting to control and shape their environment, but any activity under these auspices took place on a personal and anonymous basis. No one was attempting to make any larger structural or societal changes to

assist workers in overcoming the obstacles blocking the attainment of
their needs. The idea of having a personal problem was hidden behind
veils of secrecy and shame. The occupational environment was not being
changed; it remained the individual who had to be "fixed." Need was being
expressed, but only secretly.

"Late-stage," "forced," and "mandatory" treatment was the primary
mechanism of intervention, with Alcoholics Anonymous being the lone
significant treatment option. To an extent, AA was also an agent of social
control and resocialization, which fit into what owners and managers
desired. The non-political nature of AA aided in maintaining the status
quo and protected the workplace from having to undergo any notable or
inconvenient change. This model of mutual aid was safe for companies to
instigate and support. By focusing on individuals, it aided the employers
as much as the employees. Despite the beginnings of a new focus, the
primary motivation of these management-initiated programs continued to
be the restoration of workers to their former level of productivity, and the
creation of a more efficient workforce. However, the orientation of the
self-help movement during this period did become much less economic
and much more personal in nature. As well, mutual aid/self-help was not
only a primary resource to OAPs, but also became a major influence in its
development (Romeder, 1990).

Employee Assistance Programming

It was again the influence of Alcoholics Anonymous that served as the
catalyst for change in occupational assistance. In 1970 the United States
Congress passed the Federal Comprehensive Alcohol Abuse and Alcoholism
Prevention, Treatment and Rehabilitation Act. It was Senator Harold
Hughes, an active AA member, who spearheaded the drive for this bill,
and eventually tabled it. The Hughes Act immensely increased government
involvement in the United States in the treatment of alcoholism, producing
a variety of reforms from the decriminalization of public intoxication to
the creation of the National Institute on Alcoholism and Alcohol Abuse
(NIAAA) (Shain, 1978).

In 1971 the NIAAA, using the concept introduced by the Ontario
Addiction Research Foundation, funded and trained 120 occupational
program consultants and administrative staff. Their role was to encourage
both public and private employers in each American state to adopt an OAP.
Legislation was simultaneously introduced mandating federal government
departments and the military to introduce programming. The "Thundering
Hundred" also provided organizations with start-up grants, something that
has never occurred in Canada, setting the stage for the proliferation of

programs in the United States during the 1970s (Lotterhos, 1975; Steele, 1989; Thomlison, 1983).

Staff recruited under the program were generally not alcoholism-treatment advocates but rather professionally trained social workers and psychologists. Thus, the consultants had a bias towards training those intervening with employees to avoid identifying those in need of assistance based upon markers such as the smell of alcohol on their breath or a drunken appearance. Instead intervenors were instructed to concentrate on identifying changed work and personal behaviours of employees as markers. As concerns other than alcohol began to be consistently identified, referrals to the medical and personnel departments for assistance became fewer and were slowly replaced by a greater use of professional community-based social services (Sonnenstuhl & Trice, 1986).

By 1972 approximately 300 companies had initiated job-based alcoholism programs (Steele, 1989). In that year the NIAAA adopted the term "broadbrush" to describe an occupational assistance program with a multi-problem focus instead of one that merely assisted employees with an alcohol problem (Lotterhos, 1975). James Wrich is credited with first coining the term Employee Assistance Program, and for emphasizing the need for labour and management to work conjointly to develop a formal program policy. He advocated the implementation of systematic and coordinated procedures, including educating and training all individuals involved in assisting employees with personal problems which affected their ability to work. A key dimension in the transition from OAP to EAP was the increasing recognition of the importance of a co-operative administrative mechanism, the joint labour–management committee, which had previously been legislated in the health- and safety-field. Wrich stated that programs should no longer be unilaterally initiated by management, even if management was paying for the service. Rather, representatives of various sectors of the workplace should work together to decide what should be done to benefit the entire workforce. While designing and implementing a program took much longer using this collaborative process, it also had a greater propensity to take into consideration the needs of all employee groups (Fogarty, 1994; Wrich, 1980).

As OAP evolved into EAP, the treatment community in the United States saw an opportunity for immense increases in position, status, and revenue. This resulted in a large move into entrepreneurial private practices during the 1970s. American addiction counsellors moved away from dealing exclusively with physical health problems, and began to incorporate a variety of mental health and social problems into their medical-orientated practices. This profiteering first began to emerge in 1969 after Blue Cross and Blue Shield began to allow coverage for in-patient alcohol treatment. In 1972 Prudential Insurance became the inaugural third-party insurer to provide payments for treatment in an exclusive alcoholism recovery facility not directly affiliated with a hospital. One year later the Kemper Insurance Group, a long-time advocate of OAP, made provisions for alcoholism treatment to become a standard clause in all group policies (Kemper, 1978; McClellan, 1982a).

The rush to apply the medical-treatment model to behavioural problems, "the diseasing of America," contributed to the proliferation of third-party "helpers" in the United States. These counsellors, who generally came from outside the workplace, began to address the vast range of problems being identified by both volunteers and professionals inside the workplace, and also became an alternative to them (Favorini & Spitzer, 1993). The first documented private for-profit consulting company was inaugurated by Donald Sandin. Sandin was initially hired as an internal professional provider to assist Merrill Lynch employees in 1971. Three years later he established himself as an independent provider, and within his initial year of operation had five full-time staff servicing three organizations (ALMACA, 1983). By 1981 there were over two hundred private EAP consulting services, external to the workplace, selling employee-counselling services to companies (Sonnenstuhl & Trice, 1986). This trend came to Canada in the late 1980s with a proliferation of private practitioners in the field of occupational-assistance practice (Addiction Research Foundation, 1992; Gould & Csiernik, 1990; Vedell, 1991). Professionalism during the EAP era ran counter to the mutual-aid traditions brought to occupational assistance by AA. While there may not have been a substantive decrease in the absolute use of self-help resources, in relative terms, its role was certainly undermined during this period of privatization of the occupational-assistance field.

However, other mechanisms of mutual aid and self-help did emerge during the EAP era. Using AA as a model, labour developed its own delivery mechanism, Union Counselling. The concept of Union Counselling was originally proposed in 1942 by the Labour Division of War Production Board of the AFL-CIO, and has since been supported and promoted by the Canadian Labour Congress. This idea was congruent with labour's role in mutual aid to its membership. However, the significance of the program was not fully realized until the advent of broadbrush EAPs (Canadian Labour Congress, 1979; Miller & Metz, 1991). The United Auto Workers (UAW) and its offshoot, the Canadian Auto Workers (CAW), were not members of the AFL-CIO for a considerable period of time. As such, the UAW developed its own program similar to Union Counselling, although the focus has remained primarily upon alcohol and other psychoactive substances of abuse. Labour Substance Abuse staff are available to assist fellow union members with any drug-related problem they may have. Motivation to become a staff-person frequently arises from personal experience with and recovery from substance dependency. Substance Abuse staff also tend to have close ties to a variety of anonymous self-help groups, and in larger plants, where representatives often have their own offices, and on-site, self-help meetings are held (Masi, 1983).

As non-union and management personnel were outside the realm of the Union Counsellor movement, or tended to be reluctant to use a union-based program, a parallel stream was developed in which the term "referral agent" was used instead of Union Counsellor (Revenue Canada, 1991; Trojman, 1981; Van Halm, 1988). The responsibilities of referral agents are nearly identical to those of Union Counsellors, except that referral agents can come from any stratum of an organization's hierarchy; and, in fact, different levels are encouraged to participate so that this system has a greater resemblance to a peer-assistance program. The more generic name and the association with the broadbrush concept of EAP has also led some large unions to adopt the title "Referral Agent" rather than Union Counsellor (Canadian Union of Public Employees, 1989; Trojman, 1981).

Formal peer self-help is another form of mutual aid that became more prominent during the EAP era. The airline industry was the first to use the peer-intervention model extensively. Both the Airline Pilots (APA) and Airline Flight Attendants (AFA) Associations received demonstration funds from the NIAAA during the 1970s to initiate programs for their memberships (Molloy, 1985). This form of self-help expanded or augmented existing counselling and support services through recruiting a cadre of employees to provide mutual aid and peer support (Van Den Bergh, 1991). A chief motivation for this type of model is self-regulation, as the peer-assistance model removes the overtly and covertly coercive nature of management-initiated programming.

Of the various formats employed in delivering EAP services, the most recent to emerge has no ties to either Welfare Capitalism or OAP: the consortium. Historically EAPs have been established in large work organizations where one or more individuals operate the program on a part- or full-time basis. However, a majority of workers remains employed in organizations of 500 or less. A major issue in occupational programming over the years has been the delivery of appropriate and adequate services to smaller organizations. Traditionally, smaller companies have had insufficient resources to cope with the wide range of problems that beset all organizations and those employed by them. Motivation behind the development of consortia came initially from counsellors external to the workplace who wished to form alliances specifically with smaller businesses.

A consortium is physically located outside the organizations it serves. Program initiators retain ownership of a service that they individually could not afford, either financially or in terms of time resources, to maintain properly. Common to all consortia is the sharing of fiscal, administrative, and governing responsibilities. Representatives of the member organizations typically make decisions on issues such as staff hiring, hours of service, record keeping, and reporting through a democratic voting procedure. Some boards operate so that votes are weighted, based on each company's annual financial contribution to the consortium. In some consortia, as membership has grown it has become impractical to have 40 board members. In these instances, assignment to committees and the executive is done by means of an election, with each member organization normally assigned one vote in the electoral process.

A significant difference between consortia and other external provision models is that consortia are by design not-for-profit. Administratively, the consortium plans and directs the program in an integrated fashion. Counsellors and administrative staff are generally hired and managed through the collective auspices of the consortium. Its freestanding and independent nature are key to the growth of trust and credibility within the organizations it serves. These characteristics are also central to the safeguarding of anonymity and confidentiality, while at the same time providing a comprehensive range of clinical services to employees. Consortia also allow organizations to maintain ownership of all internal aspects of their programs, including policy and procedure creation (Csiernik, 1994).

With the move to the broadbrush approach and the emergence of EAP, the focus of workplace intervention continues to develop so that environmental factors and situations beyond the worker's immediate control are now being occasionally considered. Nevertheless, programming remains reactive in nature, continuing to individualize problems and to perceive the worker as a problem or troubled employee. EAPs can still be regarded in many respects as a management tool and as a form of social control, affecting behaviour on the job and designed to enforce compliance with management-based norms and standards (Csiernik, 1996; Pace, 1990; Yandrick, 1994). The focus of EAPs is primarily secondary prevention, the early identification of problems while the employee is still able to function in a relatively healthy manner. However, since the mid-1980s a more pro-active approach has been adopted by some organizations with a focus on primary prevention through physical health promotion initiatives.

Workplace Health Promotion Programming

Workplace health promotion programming is a combination of educational, organizational, economic, and environmental activities designed to support positive health-maintenance behaviours conducive to the well-being of employees and their families. It is about the prevention of ill health and the improvement of the quality of life, entailing both disease prevention and physical health enhancement (Parkinson, 1982; Chu, 1994). The motive behind health promotion programs is to identify, prevent, reduce, and control physiological and behavioural health risks before they develop into disabilities or premature mortality. Health promotion programs have the advantage of targeting employees who are generally functioning well, but who engage in behaviours that are likely to result in serious illnesses in the future if unchanged. Risk avoidance and risk reduction are the two prominent strategies. Risk avoidance is directed toward low-risk populations to inhibit transition to high-risk behaviours, and thereby to maintain existing levels of physical health. Risk reduction is targeted at populations already at risk and is designed to foster a transition to a lower-risk or safe status (Erfurt, Foote, & Heirich, 1992; Goodstadt, Simpson, & Loranger, 1987).

Between 53 and 93 million work days per year were lost annually during the early 1980s in Canada because of workers' illness (Air Canada, 1984; Brennan, 1985). To counter this, some organizations began examining mechanisms to promote improved employee physical health. The belief emerged that it was not only feasible to enhance worker health (and thereby produce less illness-related absenteeism), to reduce the probability of accidental injury and temporary or permanent disability, and to lower utilization of workers' compensation, health insurance, and disability insurance, but also relatively inexpensive to do so.[1] Other reported benefits that have motivated organizations to move to this phase of occupational assistance included the traditional factors: decreased employee turnover, increased productivity, increased job satisfaction, improved morale, improved public relations, monetary savings from reduced absenteeism and medical costs, and the growth of positive personal health and work practices.[2] The workplace was recognized as an excellent site for health promotion because of the amount of time people spend there, the presence of peer support, employer-provided incentives, reduced financial and time expenditures, a relatively stable and captive audience, and the increased convenience of staying on-site (Chu, 1994; Conrad, 1987; Green, 1988). Health professionals have identified the workplace as a key target for health promotion, as it is a relatively closed system with potentially powerful personal, organizational, motivational, and networking elements (Peterson, Abrams, Elder, & Beaudin, 1985).

Implementation of the inaugural health promotion program is credited to the National Cash Register Company of Dayton, Ohio, which provided a 325-acre park and a gymnasium for its employees in 1894 (Finkelstein & Frissel, 1990). This was a first-generation form of workplace health promotion, and was initiated for reasons mostly unrelated to health. Second-generation systems emerged when risk-factor identification and intervention were transported to the workplace. These programs were typically focused upon a single illness, while the next generation of health-promotion programs to emerge became more comprehensive in nature, encompassing a range of interventions for a variety of risk factors. The latest manifestation of health strategies incorporates activities, policies, and decisions that affect the health of not only employees but also family members and the community where the organization is located (Wenzel, 1994). The majority of early programming focused on the adoption or improvement of physical health-related practices such as smoking cessation, exercise and fitness, nutrition counselling and weight control, and hypertension screening; other practices included specific topics such as back care and cholesterol reduction, rather than a focus on the entire wellness continuum (Brennan, 1985; Fielding, 1984; Sonnenstuhl, 1988). However, a recent study in the province of Ontario found a dramatic growth not only in first-generation programs such as fitness (19.0 percent of workplaces in 1989 to 63.4 percent in 2003), nutrition (17.3 percent to 40.4 percent), blood pressure testing (16.4 percent to 37.4 percent), smoking cessation (29.5 percent to 51.5 percent), and weight reduction (14.7 percent to 47.5 percent), but also in some second-generation programming, featuring non-physical health initiatives such as stress management (19.3 percent to 50.5 percent) and day-care services for employees (5.9 percent to 14.4 percent) (Macdonald, Csiernik, Dooley, Durand, Rylett, Wells, & Wild, in process).

Even as mutual aid begins to shift from secondary prevention to primary prevention, the majority of self-help activity in the workplace continues to ignore the larger workplace and societal issues that underlie the need for mutual-aid initiatives. Mutual aid in the workplace, if it is to move beyond being an accessory to social control, must examine how it can assist in management issues by focusing on broader topics than personal stress management; for example, assisting in developing positive organizational change and contributing to the enhancement of workplace participation. There is a need for not only healthy workers but also for healthy workplaces.

Conclusion

During each stage of occupational assistance programming, distinctive societal influences have motivated organizations and individuals to act to improve workplace life. The industrial revolution, the introduction of Scientific Management principles, the Temperance movement, workers' compensation efforts, the 1930s depression, and the transformation of the workplace during World War II were all predominant societal factors that influenced the early evolution of occupational assistance in Canada. The formal categorization of alcoholism as a disease in the 1950s and the expansion of the disease model to encompass other psychoactive drugs also dramatically affected the development of the movement. Helping professionals, though not necessarily change agents, began to enter the workplace in larger numbers during the 1970s and 1980s. It is now widely accepted that the worksite, its organization, and the stress that work produces are major causes of illness and decreased organizational efficiency.

The drive to meet the personal needs of both helpees and helpers has been a critical motivating factor in occupational program initiation and development. However, the motivation to institute programs has not always been altruistic in nature. Self-interest, self-defence, and self-preservation have all played a part in the evolution of Canadian occupational assistance programming. One consistently positive influence throughout the entire developmental process has been mutual aid/self-help. Implicit in every self-help group is a criticism of the failures of society. The growth of mutual aid has been a response, in part, to the depersonalization of both social and work life. After a period of relatively diminished interest, mutual aid is again on the verge of being regarded as an essential feature of occupational assistance for several reasons:

i)   the increasing acceptance of mutual-aid groups by both professionals and by the general community;

ii) the vastness of issues self-help groups now encompass with treatment, primary prevention, and advocacy orientations;

iii) the fact that mutual-aid groups have negligible costs for employers who generally support, at least financially, workplace-based assistance programs.

Services flow from the way we define problems. Mutual aid evolved throughout the twentieth century from having primarily a treatment and normalization orientation to now incorporating groups with a greater emphasis upon social change. As they evolved, self-help groups helped change the focus of the occupational assistance movement from tertiary to primary prevention. There will always be a place and a need for traditional self-help groups in the workplace. However, just as mutual aid in the community evolved from Alcoholics Anonymous to consciousness-raising and advocacy groups, so self-help groups in the workplace need to move from focusing primarily upon an employee's difficulties to incorporating organizational and systems issues, which may both magnify existing problems and create new ones.

Employee participation has been hypothesized to be the key missing element in most workplace decision-making. Participation is an educative and information-sharing mechanism that breaks down traditional organizational barriers of control and decision latitude. Participation entails the creation of opportunities for workers to directly influence decisions affecting them and their work, while offering employees greater freedom of choice within the workplace environment (Briziarelli, 1989). As mutual aid/self-help is an excellent expression of consumer participation, it is an ideal model upon which to style greater workforce participation. Any success that occurs will, however, depend upon employees being given control over appropriate resources and having the authority, the ability, and the opportunity to act.

From a clinical perspective, it is time to break away from the medical model which is primarily concerned with rushing clients into treatment, and which assigns both the cause and the cure of the problem to the worker. "Victim blaming" is no longer an appropriate philosophy for occupational assistance to assert, overtly or covertly, regardless of who finances the services. Conversely, mutual aid has the potential to assist and direct the evolution of occupational assistance to the next plane of maturation, wellness programming. Active self-help groups can theoretically change the emphasis of occupational assistance from being solely worker-centered to also examining problems created by more global issues both external and internal to the workplace. Among the internal aspects are the design of the workplace and the nature of the work itself. Mutual-aid initiatives can introduce and extend social networks in the traditionally isolating workplace setting, thereby working to prevent occupational assistance from remaining a mechanism of social control. Mutual aid can be a catalyst for positive social change in the workplace. The ongoing and dramatic reductions in the welfare state along with diminishing affordable and accessible professional resources will both be critical factors that will produce increases in the need for and use of mutual aid as we move from the industrial age to the information technology-era.

Endnotes

1. Brownell, Stunkard, & McKeon, 1985; Bulaclac, 1996; Donner, 1991; Gebhardt and Crump, 1990; Shephard, Corey, Renzland, & Cox, 1982; Sipkoff & Oss, 1993.

2.   Patton, 1991; Peepre, 1980; Renner, 1987; Roman & Blum, 1988; Shehadeh
     & Shain, 1990; Yardley, 1985.

References

Addiction Research Foundation. (1992). *Resource directory to Employee Assistance
     Programs*. Toronto: Addiction Research Foundation.

Air Canada. (1984). *Air Canada's health promotion program*. Toronto: Air Canada
     Medical Services Department.

Allen, J. (1966). *The company town in the American west*. Norman, Oklahoma:
     University of Oklahoma Press.

Allen, R. (1971). *The social passion*. Toronto: University of Toronto Press.

ALMACA. (1983). Pioneer of the private consultants. *Labour–Management
     Alcoholism Journal* 12(6), 181–205.

Baxter, J. (1984) Employee Assistance Programs in historical perspective:
     The meddling of economics and human concerns. In R. Thoreson & E.
     Hosokawa (eds.), *Employee Assistance Programs in higher education*. Springfield:
     Charles C. Thomas.

Bennett, K. (1975*). Development of Industrial Alcoholism Programs in Hamilton,
     Ontario*. Hamilton: Addiction Research Foundation.

Boyer, C. (1983). *The Myth of American city planning*. Cambridge: MIT Press.

Brandes, S. (1976*). American Welfare Capitalism, 1880–1940*. Chicago: University
     of Chicago Press.

Brennan, A. (1985). Health and fitness boom moves into corporate America.
     EAP Digest 6(1), 29–36.

Briziarelli, L. (1989). Worker's participation: A key to health promotion at the
     workplace. *Health promotion in the working world*. Federal Centre for Health
     Education. New York: Springer-Verlag.

Brownell, K., Stunkard, A., & McKeon, P. (1985) Weight reduction at the work
     site: A promise partially fulfilled. *American Journal of Psychiatry* 142(1), 47–
     51.

Bulaclac, M. (1996). A worksite wellness program. *Nursing Management* 27(12),
     19–21.

Caldwell, J. (1977). *A Study of EAPs in Ontario*. Toronto: ARF.

Canadian Labour Congress. (1979). *A guide for developing a Union Counsellor program
     for local labour councils*. Ottawa: CLC/United Way.

Canadian Union of Public Employees. (1989). *Helping ourselves: Employee
     Assistance Programs*. Ottawa.

Carter, I. (1977). Social work in industry: A history and a viewpoint. *Social
     Thought* 3(1), 7–17.

Chu, C. (1994) An integrated approach to workplace health promotion. In C.
     Chu and R. Simpson (eds.), *Ecological Public Health: From Vision to Practice*.
     Toronto: ParticipACTION.

Conrad, P. (1987). Wellness in the workplace: Potentials and pitfalls of worksite health promotion. *Milbank Quarterly* 65(2), 255–275.

Corneil, W. (1984). History, philosophy and objectives of an Employee Recovery Program. In W. Albert, B. Boyle, & C. Ponee (eds.), *EAP Orientation: Volume II—Important concepts.* Toronto: Addiction Research Foundation.

Csiernik, R. (1994). Employee Assistance consortia: Developing a research agenda. *Employee Assistance Quarterly* 10(2), 19–35.

Csiernik, R. (1996). Occupational social work: From social control to social assistance? *The Social Worker* 64 (3), 67–74.

Donner, B. (1991). Achieving a healthier workplace. *Health Promotion* 29(3), 2–6, 24.

Dunkin, W. (1982). A brief history of Employee Alcoholism/Assistance Programs. *Labour–Management Alcoholism Journal* 11(5), 165–168.

Erfurt, J., Foote, A., & Heirich, M. (1992). Integrating Employee Assistance and wellness: Current and future core technologies of a megabrush program. *Journal of Employee Assistance Research* 1(1), 1–31.

Favorini, A. & Spitzer, K. (1993). The emergence of external Employee Assistance Programs: Report of a survey and identification of trends. *Journal of Employee Assistance Research* 2(1), 23–35.

Fielding, J. (1984). *Corporate Health Management.* Don Mills: Addison-Wesley.

Finkelstein, D. & Frissel, S.(1990). The systems/integrated approach to quality and cost-effective care. *Employee Assistance Quarterly* 6(1), 25–44.

Fogarty, B. (1994). AFL-CIO has history of helping employees tackle substance abuse. *EAPA Exchange* 24(1), 37.

Garner, J. (1984). *The model company town.* Amherst: University of Massachusetts.

Gartner, A. & Riessman, F. (1977). *Self-help in the human services.* Washington: Jossey-Bass.

Gebhardt, D. & Crump, C. (1990) Employee fitness and wellness programs in the workplace. *American Psychologist* 45(2), 262–272.

Germain, C. (1973). An ecological perspective in casework practice. *Social Casework* 54(6), 323–330.

Germain, C. (1978). General systems theory and ego psychology: An ecological perspective. *Social Service Review* 52(4), 535–550.

Germain, C. (1979). *Social work practice, people and environments.* New York: Columbia University Press.

Goodstadt, M., Simpson, R., & Loranger, P. (1987). Health promotion: A conceptual integration. *American Journal of Health Promotion* 1(1), 58–63.

Googins, B. & Godfrey, J. (1987). *Occupational Social Work.* Englewood Cliffs: Prentice Hall.

Gosden, P. (1973). *Self-help: Voluntary associations in the 19th Century.* London: B.T. Batsford Limited.

Gould, A. & Csiernik, R. (1990). *EAP Service Providers' Guide*. Hamilton: Employee Assistance Program Council of Hamilton-Wentworth.

Green, K.L. (1988). Issues of control and responsibility in workers' health. *Health Education Quarterly* 15(4), 473–486.

Haney, W. (1979). *Communication and interpersonal relations*. Georgetown: Irwin-Dorsey.

Juran, J.M., Gryna, F., Jr., & Bingham, R.S. (1951). *Quality control handbook*. Toronto: McGraw-Hill.

Katz, A. & Bender, E. (1976). *The strength in us*. New York: New Viewpoints.

Kealey, G. & Palmer, B. (1982). *Dreaming of what might be: The Knights of Labour in Ontario, 1880–1900*. New York: Cambridge University Press.

Kerans, P., Dorver, G., & Williams, D. (1988). *Welfare and worker participation*. New York: St. Martin's Press.

Kemper, J., Jr. (1978). The Kemper Program. *Labour–Management Alcoholism Journal* 7(4), 3–28.

Lindop, S. (1975). Three Canadian industrial alcoholism programs. In R. Williams & G. Moffat (eds.), *Occupational Alcoholism Programs*. Springfield: Charles C. Thomas.

Lotterhos, J. (1975). Historical and sociological perspectives of alcohol-related problems. In R. Williams & G. Moffat (eds.), *Occupational Alcoholism Programs*. Springfield: Charles C. Thomas.

Macdonald, S., Csiernik, R., Dooley, S., Durand, P., Rylett, M., Wells, S., & Wild, C. (in process). *Trends and regional differences across Canada in worksite programs to address substance abuse: 1989–2003*.

Mackintosh, M. (1939). Workmen's compensation in Canada. *International Labour Review* 40, 1–31.

Masi, D. (1983). *Human services in industry*. Toronto: Lexington Books.

Masi, D. (1984). *Designing Employee Assistance Programs*. New York: American Management Association.

Massey, M. & Csiernik, R. (1997). Community development in EAP: The Employee Assistance Program Council of Hamilton-Wentworth. *Employee Assistance Quarterly* 12(3), 35–46.

McClellan, K. (1982a). An overview of occupational alcoholism issues for the 80's. *Journal of Drug Education* 12, 1–27.

McClellan, K. (1982b). The consortium approach to EAP services. *EAP Digest* 2(2), 33–35.

McGilly, F. (1985). American historical antecedents to industrial social work. *Social Work Papers of the School of Social Work, University of Southern California* 19, 1–13.

McGregor, D. (1960). *The human side of enterprise*. New York: McGraw Hill.

Miller, R. & Metz, G. (1991). Union Counselling as peer assistance. *Employee Assistance Quarterly* 6(4), 1–21.

Molloy, D. (1985). Peer referral. In S. Klareich, J. Francek, & C.E. Moore (eds.), *The Human Resources Handbook*. Toronto: Prager Press.

Pace, E. (1990). Peer Employee Assistance Programs for nurses. *Perspectives on Addictions Nursing* 1(4), 3–7.

Parkinson, R.S. (1982). *Managing health promotion in the workplace*. Palo Alto: Mayfield.

Patton, J. (1991). Work-site health promotion: An economic model. *Journal of Occupational Medicine* 33(8), 868–873.

Peepre, M. (1980). The Canadian employee fitness and lifestyle project. *Athletic Purchasing and Facilities*, December 1–8.

Petersen, K. (1987). *Company town: Potlatch, Idaho and the Potlatch Lumber Company*. Pullman, Washington: Washington State University Press.

Peterson, G., Abrams, D., Elder, J., & Beaudin, P. (1985). Professional versus self-help weight loss at the worksite: The challenge of making a public health impact. *Behaviour Therapy* 16, 213–221.

Popple, P. (1981). Social work practice in business and industry, 1875–1930. *Social Service Review* 55, 257–269.

Presnall, L. (1981) *Occupational counselling and referral systems*. Salt Lake City: Utah Alcoholism Foundation.

Preston, H. & Bierman, M. (1985). An insurance company EAP. *EAP Digest* 6(1), 21–28.

Renner, J. (1987). Wellness programs: An investment in cost containment. *EAP Digest* 7(3), 49–53.

Revenue Canada. (1991). *Referral agent training manual*. Ottawa.

Rimlinger, G. (1983). Capitalism and human rights. *Daedalus* Fall, 51–79.

Robin, M. (1968). *Radical Politics and Canadian Labour*. Kingston: Industrial Relations Centre.

Robinson, D. & Henry, S. (1977). *Self-help and health*. Bungay: Chaucer Press.

Robinson, I. (1962). *New industrial towns on Canada's resource frontier*. Chicago: University of Chicago Press.

Romeder, J. (1990). *The self-help way: Mutual aid and health*. Ottawa: Canadian Council on Social Development.

Scanlon, W. (1986). *Alcoholism and drug abuse in the workplace*. Toronto: Praeger Press.

Scheinberg, S. (1986). *Employers and reformers: The development of corporation labour policy, 1990–1940*. New York: Garland.

Shain, M. (1978). *Occupational programming: The state of the art as seen through literature reviews and current studies*. Toronto: Addiction Research Foundation.

Shain, M. & Groeneveld, J. (1980). *Employee Assistance Programs: Philosophy, theory and practice.* Toronto: Lexington Books.

Shehadeh, V. & Shain, M. (1990*). Influences on wellness in the workplace: A multivariate approach.* Ottawa: Health and Welfare Canada.

Shephard, R., Corey, P., Renzland, P., & Cox, M. (1982). The influence of an employee fitness and lifestyle modification program upon medical care costs. *Canadian Journal of Public Health* 73(4), 259–263.

Sipkoff, M. & Oss, M. (1993). Trends in stress-related Workers' Compensation claims. *EAP Digest* 13(3), 28–30.

Sonnenstuhl, W. (1988). Contrasting Employee Assistance, health promotion, and quality of work life programs and their effects on alcohol abuse and dependence. *Journal of Applied Behavioural Science* 24(4), 347–363.

Sonnenstuhl, W. & Trice, H. (1986). *Strategies for Employee Assistance Programs: The crucial balance.* New York: ILR Press.

Steele, P. (1989). A history of job-based alcoholism programs: 1955–1972. *Journal of Drug Issues* 19(4), 511–532.

Straussner, S. (1989). Occupational social work today: An overview. *Employee Assistance Quarterly*, 5(1), 1–17.

Thomlison, R. (1983). Industrial social work: Perspectives and issues. In R. Thomlinson (ed.), *Perspectives on industrial social work.* Toronto: Family Service Canada.

Torjman, S. (1981). *A training course for EAP Referral Agents.* Ottawa: Health and Welfare Canada.

Trice, H. & Schonbrunn, M. (1988). A history of job-based alcoholism programs, 1900–1955. In F. Dickman, B.R. Challenger, W. Emener, & W. Hutchinson, Jr. (eds.), *Employee Assistance Programs: A basic text.* Springfield, Illinois: Charles C. Thomas.

Trice, H. & Sonnenstuhl, W. (1985). Contributions of AA to Employee Assistance Programs. *Employee Assistance Quarterly* 1(1), 7–31.

Van Den Bergh, N. (1991). Workplace mutual aid and self-help: Invaluable resources for EAPs. *Employee Assistance Quarterly* 6(3), 1–20.

Van Halm, R. (1988). Out of the woods. *Occupational Health and Safety Canada* 4(6), 22–29.

Vedell, J. (1991). Counselling at family services: Historical snapshots. *Family Focus* 15(1), 4.

Wenzel, E. (1994). Conceptual issues in worksite health promotion. In C. Chu & R. Simpson (eds.), *Ecological public health: From vision to practice.* Toronto: ParticipACTION.

Wilson, B. (1957). *Alcoholics Anonymous comes of age.* New York: Harper & Brothers.

Windsor, R. & Bartlett, E. (1984). Employee self-help smoking cessation programs: A review of the literature. *Health Education Quarterly* 11(4), 349–359.

Wrich, J. (1980). *The Employee Assistance Program*. Centre City: Hazelden.

Yandrick, R. (1994). Has the core technology become an anachronism? *EAPA Exchange* 24(2), 6–9.

Yardley, J. (1985). Benefits/costs of employee fitness, recreation and assistance programs: Is it worthwhile for your company? Paper delivered at *Fitness: A Practical Approach in the Workplace Conference,* Jordan Station, Ontario, March 7.

Zahavi, G. (1988). Workers, managers, and Welfare Capitalism: The shoeworkers and tanners of Endicott Johnson, 1890–1950. Chicago: University of Illinois Press.

3

Disability Management
in the Canadian Context

Tony Fasulo and Sara Martel

Introduction

Like any social institution, Canadian work-life has undergone significant
instrumental changes since industrialization and the beginnings of private
industry, organized labour, mass production, and management practices.
While the nature of the current and proceeding period in Canadian
labour history has yet to be fully determined, the authors believe it may
be distinguished from previous eras by its focus on health and well-being
within the workplace. This is true in terms not just of occupational health
services, but also of disability management and Employee Assistance
Programming (EAP).

The existence of disability-management programming signals a changed
perspective on the labourer and the workplace from the days when
employee health was simply not on the map of management initiative. It
is difficult to imagine employee health and rehabilitation integrated directly
into management policy in any workplace typical of early industrial society,
where a Scientific Management and a "worker as machine" mentality
predominated. We certainly are not suggesting that a workers' "utopia" has
since emerged: we are well aware of the pressures facing workers today in
a global work-world of high competition, vast markets, increased labour
pools, and fear of redundancy. Rather, during the last half of the twentieth-
century and the beginning of the twenty-first, there has developed a
discourse and practice around employee wellness, vocational rehabilitation,
and labour–management initiatives where none had previously existed
(Quinn, 1995; Shrey, 2000; Smith, 1997).

The result of this development is the incorporation of disability,
management practice into the workplace as an initiative of the employer,

rather than, at most, offering off-site rehabilitation and (at the least) treating employees as disposable assets. Today disability management is seen as a workplace necessity that reduces costs, increases productivity, and reflects an overall understanding of the value healthy employees bring to any successful business. As more employers understand the importance of human capital, disability management provides them with the tools to maintain a healthier workplace and to maximize their employees' productivity. While the advantage to employers is undeniable, the benefits of disability management for employees likewise cannot be overlooked. Progressive disability management is not a method of labour control, or of social control, but rather a rehabilitation and health promotion tool.[1]

Disability management and EAP offer many of the same advantages to both employers and employees, and it is this commonality and the potential partnership it can build that warrant attention here. This chapter will familiarize readers with the history and current form of disability management. It will also illustrate how disability management and EAP can come together to take workplace environments to the next phase in labour history: when all workplaces have fully integrated programs incorporating EAP and disability management to create a culture of workplace wellness.

A Brief History of Disability Management

It is notoriously difficult to define "disability management"; this difficulty is in fact a recurring theme in prefaces on the subject. Disability management escapes concise definition due both to the diversity of disciplines it incorporates, and to the functions it encompasses. Operationally, disability management can be defined as "a proactive process that minimizes the impact of an impairment, resulting from injury, illness, or disease on the individual's capacity to participate competitively in the work environment" (Shrey, 1995). Conceptually, however, it encompasses a much broader concept of wellness in the workplace, one which continues to evolve and expand.

The beginnings of disability management are largely marked by the relocation and expansion of external rehabilitation services into on-site vocational rehabilitation policy, practice, and training. In Canada, the National Institute of Disability Management and Research (NIDMAR) has shaped these roots since its formation in 1994. NIDMAR arose from the co-operation of MacMillan Bloedel Limited, IWA-CANADA, the Disabled Workers Foundation of Canada, formerly called the Disabled Forestry Workers Foundation of Canada and the Communications, Energy, and Paperworkers Union of Canada (CEP), commonly referred to as the Canadian Paperworkers Union (Riessner, 1995). Together these groups set out to explore and resolve issues around disability in the workplace, including the management of ever-increasing disability costs and the challenge of returning disabled employees to work in a physically healthy manner. Prior to this work done in the mid-1990s, disability costs were simply accepted and absorbed as inevitable business expenditure, and absenteeism was seen as an issue relating to problem employees, rather than to overall workplace strategy.

Today NIDMAR acts as an education and training centre for the disability-management model these initial collectives eventually developed after several international studies, interviews, worksite visits, and model analyses. The NIDMAR (2003) website states, "As an education, training and research organization, NIDMAR's primary focus is the implementation of workplace-based reintegration programs which international research has proven is the most effective way of restoring and maintaining workers' abilities, while reducing the costs of disability for workers, employers, government and insurance carriers." As a resource for the implementation of disability-management programs, NIDMAR's value is its focus on a joint labour–management, peer-consensus implementation. The NIDMAR model espouses education for and support from all workplace groups. Fortunately, support can be achieved due to disability management's mutual benefit to both labour and management, allowing businesses to include this initiative equally in both their economic and health-promotion strategies. It could be argued that this flexible duality is in fact the driving force behind the success of disability management in Canadian businesses.

The story of disability management is an unfinished one, however, as program models continue to develop and goals expand. Increasingly, the focus on individual injuries and disabilities is broadening, and disability-management strategies are evolving to meet new challenges and provide more comprehensive solutions. We will explore these responses in the following section, putting a form and function to them by way of an introduction to the actual shape of contemporary disability-management programs.

Implementing a Disability-Management Program

We discussed above how disability management is difficult to define in any singular form. Even as the operational term remains the same, disability-management programs can take on a number of different shapes when actually realized within the workplace (Pransky, Shaw, Franche, & Clarke, 2004). The outline of disability-management programs we provide here, therefore, is inevitably coloured by the specific approach we take as disability-management professionals. Most prominently, this approach is characterized by a focus on ability, as opposed to disability. At its best, we believe disability management actually takes on the form of ability management; that is, a more comprehensive approach to preventing injury, educating and training all employees on health and safety in the workplace, prioritizing early intervention, aiming for healthy return to work or accommodating current work abilities and expanding the scope of disabilities dealt with within the disability-management mandate. We discuss below the components of a disability-management program as informed by this approach.

Identifying Disability-Management Needs and Corporate Culture

One of the first tasks in establishing a disability-management program is getting to know the workplace itself: what plan design is currently in place? How many employees are there? Where are the disability-management weaknesses? Where are the strengths? What are the main cost sources? All of these questions and others can be answered with a comprehensive disability-management audit based on the NIDMAR audit model. In essence, an audit is a report card grading an organization's current disability-management practices and procedures. The grades are derived from information gathered on the organization through interviews with different staff and departments, case-activity reviews, and formal process analysis. An examination of the data provides an accurate image of the disability-management deficiencies and achievements; this information can be used to create a tailored program for the organization if it wishes.

A disability-management program designed to reflect the unique corporate culture of a specific workplace is much more likely to meet with long-term success. The advantage of learning the business's character is twofold. In addition to the benefit of customizing a program to meet specific needs, this process allows the provider to get to know the workplace groups and build the support for the program that is so integral to success. Disability management must not only involve the injured employee and his/her direct supervisor, but all employees, local/senior management, union representation, occupational health and safety teams, and the EAP. The audit helps identify how these groups currently participate in disability-management practices, if at all, as well as the kind of training required to have them functionally and accountably involved once the formal program is established.

Creating a Disability-Management Team

The next phase of constructing a solid disability-management program within the workplace is to assemble a disability-management team whose organization best responds to the issues identified by the audit. Regardless of the specific issues, the disability-management team will certainly include case managers, sometimes referred to as disability-management consultants, who are on the front-line of the disability-management process. In general terms, case managers liaise between injured or ill employees, managers, labour representatives, and treating physicians. Essentially the case manager contacts the employee upon absence, then gathers medical information related to the absence. If the medical information from the treating physician does not correspond to the reasons given for absence, the case manager can coordinate further independent medical examinations to determine the physical or mental barriers to work. While the case manager does not reveal the employee's medical diagnosis to the employer for confidentiality reasons, he/she does share the employee's functional capacity in order to let the employer know the expected return-to-work schedule.

Case managers are absolutely critical to the overall disability-management process. Their contact with the employee and employer can dismantle or advance the process based on the trust and co-operation established, the communication fostered, and the appropriateness of the recommendations they make for treatment or return to work. The case-management team can consist of a variety of healthcare professionals, including certified kinesiologists, occupational therapists, vocational rehabilitation specialists, registered social workers, registered nurses, and other related helping professionals.

Not all disability-management programs have the same team structure. Many are extensive, offering coordinators, quality-assurance personnel, account managers, and health specialists, while others consist mainly of the case managers with a few additional administrative support positions. What is most important in putting this team together, in addition to making sure it suits the organization's needs and goals, is ensuring that both labour and management interests are reflected in the structure and available resources. This best occurs through the creation of a Joint Labour–Management Committee, which is what should also occur within an organization's EAP structure. This internal team is responsible for ensuring that the disability-management program addresses the needs and concerns of the various workplace groups. The feasibility of a Joint Labour–Management Committee in disability management, like in EAP, depends upon the organization's size and resources. If it is not possible to formalize such a committee, a sense of commitment to labour–management co-operation through consistent, open communication between all workplace groups and the disability-management provider, as well as ongoing training on everyone's individual roles/responsibilities, should be both encouraged and developed.

Developing a Communication Strategy

Disability management can move forward only when all workplace groups understand its function and co-operate in reaching its goals of decreasing absences, preventing injury and/or illness, returning employees to work if/when possible, and promoting overall health and wellness in the workplace. This foundational understanding rarely occurs without effort, given that managers and employees alike are often unfamiliar with disability management as a general term, let alone with their new roles and responsibilities within the process. Solid communication strategies begin with informational material for employees, and education/training initiatives for management, unions, and other groups involved. This initial training should be followed by frequent and consistent communication between the provider and the groups in respect of claim activity, program progress, and ongoing education and discussion on specific issues that may arise. Finally, comprehensive statistical reporting is important, so program progress is tracked, trends are identified, statistics are analysed, and the path of long-term program goals is clarified. Together these ongoing communication initiatives create informed support as well as accountability for individual staff roles and responsibilities within the process (Pransky, Shaw, Franche, and Clarke, 2004).

The Next Step in Disability Management

The above discussion introduces the basic function and forms of disability-management programs. Of course, additional elements and specific approaches must be added to this frame before the image of a truly effective disability management program emerges. We focus on two such characteristics here, which we are highlighting given their positive contributions to the function of EAP.

Beyond the medical model to comprehensive disability management

As a practice, disability management has moved away from a strictly medical model that assumes a direct link between the employee's medical impairment and the disability or inability to work productively. The medical model positions employees to focus on their disability, encouraging them to prove that the impairment substantiates their inability to work or necessitates the receipt of benefits. What has developed since, and what we personally advocate as professionals, is a focus on ability versus disability, as well as a more holistic approach to disability management that looks at the individual's personal, social, psychological, professional, and physical health in relation to their absence.

This development is particularly important in light of the findings in Watson Wyatt's *Staying@Work 2002/2003* study, which indicates that psychological conditions are a leading cause of short-term and long-term disability costs. Disability management has incorporated psychological case management in the past, but case managers and employers have been slow to effectively target psychological issues due to the barriers built and maintained by the medical model (Olsheski, Rosenthal, & Hamilton, 2002). To maximize the disability management and EAP partnership, disability-management providers must develop more direct programs and services to deal with psychological cases, in order to decrease the risk of losing employees after the conclusion of their EAP sessions. The kinds of services, supports, or interventions we are advocating here would move beyond traditional assessment and case management and become more objective, comprehensive, and sensitive to the cognitive and behavioural elements of disability. Furthermore, these services and interventions would identify the underlying causes of certain impairments, such as workplace tensions, personal obstacles, alcohol abuse, lack of job suitability, and related issues, which otherwise can go unaddressed, even if they are detected.

Objectivity in a third-party provider
Disability management must be objective in all its capacities, from the beginning to the end of the process. Some perceive disability-management providers as working primarily in the interests of the employer, largely because the employer hires and pays the provider. Successful disability management aims for timely return to work, even on gradual, modified, or alternate terms, but only if it is possible for the employee to return in a healthy manner. Sending employees to work when they are not physically or mentally capable of doing so simply increases the likelihood of re-injury, prolonged disability, and decreased productivity, while also creating a host of liability issues. Disability management obviously aims to reduce the employer's disability-related costs, but this is never done without regard for the employees' health. In fact, if it is achieved without regard for employee well-being, the disability-management provider is simply not doing its job.

Objectivity is dually important for disability management in regards to the EAP partnership as it allows for assessment that is not structured to prove the ability or inability to work, but rather to identify and legitimate broader issues that are barriers to work. This kind of assessment, along with the comprehensive case management described above, further supports the work done by EAP professionals: it allows the disability-management provider to remain open to a range of additional concerns that might otherwise be dismissed if the sole objective were to assess ability to work based on a subjective, economic agenda (Brines, Salazar, Graham, & Pergola, 1999).

Disability Management and Employee Assistance Programming

The ultimate goal of combining EAP and disability-management efforts is to maximize both their capacities to keep or return employees to full health and productive, suitable work. There are two points within a wellness strategy that are particularly relevant to this goal: early intervention and health promotion/disability prevention.

Early intervention

NIDMAR has produced some striking numbers on the value of early intervention: "Research and practical experience have shown that for employees who have incurred a disability: there is only a 50 percent chance they will return to work after a six month absence; declining to a 20 percent chance after a one year absence, and reduced to a 10 percent chance after a two year absence" (Riessner, 1995). The obvious point here is that a disability-management program is most likely to meet with successful return to work rates when the process begins immediately upon illness or injury.

EAP discourse also includes the idea of early intervention in the context of addressing issues before they develop into larger, chronic problems. Within EAP, early intervention manifests itself through the encouragement of self-referral and the provision of short-term counselling while the employee is still at work. In many ways, Employee Assistance Programming is quintessentially an early-intervention strategy for disability management as it allows the employee to seek help before the issue in question results in disability. The fact remains, however, that despite these efforts, many psychosocial issues lead to time off work, making the disability-management process indispensable. This transitional point between using the EAP and leaving work is a crucial time within which both the EAP and the disability-management team could partner so as to strengthen early-intervention efforts (Smith, 1997).

While EAP providers cannot give disability-management case managers specific information on employees due to confidentiality issues, they can generate and share overall trends and statistics. These statistics could allow disability-management case managers to prepare for certain types of disability without the EAP disclosing any identifiable information. For instance, if the EAP reports that a significant percentage of self-referrals is dealing with depression-related issues, disability-management case managers will know ahead of time to look for this kind of disability, target assessment, and identify root issues, medical conditions, relationships and tensions, particularly if the workplace itself is the primary stressor. The result can be minimizing both misguided case management and unnecessary time-off, and improving the likelihood of return to work. Immediate identification of the disability source is particularly helpful with respect to psychosocial disabilities, as the root causes are often difficult to objectively assess without addressing issues within the individual's personal, social, and work life.

Further, if a given department has a high rate of one psychosocial condition specifically, the disability-management provider, alone or in co-operation with the EAP, has the ability to explore workplace dynamics and job-related stressors that may lead to a detrimental environment. The ability to understand and affect relationships and job elements relating to illness and impairment is a fundamental benefit of disability management. It is also another reason that disability-management providers must maintain complete objectivity. Progressive disability management allows for a critical approach to the workplace, allowing the freedom to openly explore and address negative dynamics and relationships. This inside-out approach can assist in effecting change within the workplace itself, creating a healthy culture as opposed to merely rehabilitating individual disabilities in an isolated manner.

Health promotion and disability prevention
While it is inevitable that some employees will face absences due to disability, it remains important to promote health and prevention throughout the workplace. Again, disability-management providers and EAP professionals can pool their resources to create very effective educational material and/ or workshops for labour and management, from both a counselling and case-management perspective. A clear image of health and prevention can emerge from coupling the psychosocial angle EAP takes with the information on functional capacity, ergonomic safety, and so on, which disability-management professionals are able to provide. Together, this kind of insight creates a pro-active approach to workplace wellness that does not wait until employees are disabled before involving the employee and employer in an overall wellness strategy.

Health promotion and disability prevention, as well as early intervention, are all part of an integrated way of dealing with wellness in the workplace. Essentially we are proposing that disability-management providers, EAP professionals and peer supports, occupational health and safety committees, and other programs work together towards the same goal in an integrated manner, rather than working in isolation alongside one another. This is the difference between having one program focused on disabled workers, and a system of integrated programs in a workplace culture with a central focus on wellness. We believe the future of disability management includes this form of integration, which employers will initiate as an integral facet of intelligent business policy and practice, as well as a responsibility they have to their employees.

Conclusion: Challenges and Risks

Among the most serious risks to consider is the breach of boundaries. EAP counselling can be a very safe but still potentially fragile space for employees. It is imperative to maintain the boundaries between this space and any other within the workplace, including the disability-management process. It is important to understand that by "integration" we are not suggesting all workplace groups will amalgamate into a single indistinguishable process. We mean, rather, that all workplace groups should maintain their individual functions and integrity, while recognizing that they all focus on employee health and can co-operate to achieve shared goals. In other words, EAPs, disability management, occupational health and safety personnel, and all others would serve as individual but mutually interested components of a single wellness-focused mechanism. For this structure to succeed, employees must be educated about the functions of each element and understand their role within the elements. At the same time, it is also be the employer's responsibility to ensure these elements are working for its employees, constantly balancing the bottom line with employee interest.

Another potential challenge is to alter the perception held by employees, union representatives, EAP, or others that disability-management providers work primarily for the employer, with the narrow mandate of cost control at any expense—even the expense of employee health or safety. The reduction of disability-related costs is unequivocally a part of disability management (Burton & Conti, 2000; Mobley, Linz, Shukla, Breslin, & Deng, 2000). Cost reduction, however, should not occur at the expense of employee health. Rather, disability costs can be managed by preventing and educating about injury and illness that become disabilities, promoting healthy workplaces to avoid work-related impairment, assessing and identifying the more complex reasons for absence outside of direct physical disability, opening discussion on workplace tensions and stressors, intervening early in a claim with effective case management to ensure the employee is getting proper rehabilitative treatment, and designing appropriate return-to-work programs so employees get back to work in a healthy yet timely manner (Caulfield, 1996; Shrey, 1996).

The developments we have outlined thus far will not be expeditiously implemented nor perfected in one solid phase. Rather, the EAP/disability management partnership is one that will come to fruition through much negotiation, communication, and ongoing efforts by all involved. Once the above benefits are realized and brought together with the invaluable work of EAP, labour environments across Canada have the potential to meet with greatly improved wellness standards within employee-positive workplace cultures.

Endnotes

1. Boseman, 2001; Tate, Habeck, Rochelle, & Schwartz, 1986; Williams & Westmorland, 2002.

References

Boseman, J. (2001). Disability management: Application of a nurse-based model in a large corporation. *American Association of Occupational Health Nurses Journal* 49(4), 176–186.

Brines, J., Salazar, M., Graham, K., & Pergola, T. (1999). Return to work experience of injured workers in a case management program. *American Association of Occupational Health Nurses Journal* 47(8), 365–372.

Burton, W. & Conti, D. (2000). Disability management: Corporate medical department management of employee health and productivity. *Journal of Occupational and Environmental Medicine* 42 (10), 1006–1012.

Caufield, C. (1996). Partners in health: A case study of a comprehensive disability management program. *Health Management Forum* 9(2), 36–43.

Mobley, E., Linz, D., Shukla, R., Breslin, R., & Deng, C. (2000). Disability case management: An impact assessment in an automotive manufacturing organization. *Journal of Occupational and Environmental Medicine* 42(6), 597–602.

National Institute of Disability Management and Research. (2003). http:// www.nidmar.ca/about/about_institute/institute_info.asp

Olshesik, J., Rosenthal, D., & Hamilton, M. (2002). Disability management and psychosocial rehabilitation: Considerations for integration. *Work: A Journal of Prevention, Assessment, and Rehabilitation* 19(1), 63–70.

Pransky, G., Shaw, W., Franche, R., & Clarke, A. (2004). Disability prevention and communication among workers, physicians, employers, and insurers—current models and opportunities for improvement. *Disability and Rehabilitation* 26 (11), 625–634.

Quinn, P. (1995). Social work and disability management policy: Yesterday, today and tomorrow. *Social Work in Health Care* 20(3), 67–82.

Riessner, S. (1995) *Disability management in the workplace: A guide to establishing a joint workplace program.* Port Alberni, British Colombia: The National Institute of Disability Management and Research.

Shrey, D. (1995). Worksite disability management and industrial rehabilitation. In D. Shrey & M. Lacerte (eds.), *Principles & practices of disability management in industry.* Winter Park, Florida: GR Press.

Shrey, D. (1996). Disability management in industry: The new paradigm in injured worker rehabilitation. *Disability and Rehabilitation* 18(8), 408–414.

Shrey, D. (2000). Worksite disability management model for effective return-to-work planning. *Occupational Medicine* 15(4), 789–801.

Smith, D. (1997). Implementing disability management: A review of basic concepts and essential components. *Employee Assistance Quarterly* 12(4), 37–50.

Tate, D., Habeck, R., & Schwartz, G. (1986). Disability management: A comprehensive framework for prevention and rehabilitation in the workplace. *Rehabilitation Literature* 47(9–10), 230–235.

Watson Wyatt. (2003). *Staying@Work 2002/2003: Building on Disability Management.* Toronto: Watson Wyatt.

Williams, R. & Westmorland, M. (2002). Perspectives on workplace disability management: A review of the literature. *Work: A Journal of Prevention, Assessment, and Rehabilitation* 19 (1), 87–93.

4

Drug Testing in the Workplace:
Issues, Answers, and
the Canadian Perspective

Scott Macdonald

Introduction

Drug testing is a process that detects metabolites from illicit and prescription drugs. Drug tests are generally conducted to detect five classes of drug metabolites: cannabis, cocaine, opiates, benzodiazepines, and amphetamines. The most common type of drug testing in the workplace is urinalysis. However, urinalysis tests cannot determine whether someone is currently under the influence of drugs; they can only assess whether a person was exposed to drugs in the past, and even this varies as drug metabolites are eliminated from the body at different rates. Testing of blood, hair, or saliva is also possible; however, given the various technical and ethical limitations, these approaches are much less common. By contrast, the breathalyser is used to detect alcohol levels in the blood, and these levels correlate strongly with degree of impairment.

In the past two decades, urinalysis testing of employees has increased dramatically in North America. What are the reasons for this increase and why have companies adopted drug-testing programs? Is drug use actually a major cause of workplace accidents and injuries? How effective are drug-testing programs in the workplace and are they justifiable in the Canadian workplace? What do authoritative institutions in Canada have to say about the advisability of drug testing in the workplace? These important questions will be addressed in this chapter.

History and Rationale for Drug Testing

The majority of growth in the drug-testing arena occurred after the signing of a United States Federal Executive Order in 1986 mandating drug testing for some federal government employees and those in the safety-sensitive transportation area. In 1988, the Drug-Free Workplace Act was signed. This Act required American companies with large federal contracts to promote a drug-free working environment. Mandatory guidelines were subsequently introduced for government employees and several Supreme Court decisions affirmed the legality of drug testing in the workplace. The proportion of companies with drug-testing programs in the United States likely peaked in the mid-1990s, with 52 percent of US companies having some form of drug testing in 1991 but only 47 percent reporting using this procedure in 2000 (American Management Association, 2000).

Although the executive order mandated drug testing and paved the way for American companies to adopt drug testing, the research and rationale for drug testing were not well articulated. The underlying assumption is that employees who use drugs on or off the job tend to be less reliable, less productive, prone to greater absenteeism, and pose a serious health and safety threat to members of the public. Drug testing in the workplace was also justified as a means of *reducing drug use in society* through deterrence (Executive Order, 1986). Simultaneously, the United States' "War on Drugs," using traditional criminal justice approaches to reduce drug use, had largely failed to alleviate the problem (MacCoun & Reuter, 2001), with survey studies indicating that 70 percent of drug users had jobs. Proponents argue that if drug-using employees could be targeted in the workplace, drug use in society could be substantially reduced. Therefore, the identification of drug users in the workplace, where traditional safeguards of civil liberties could be bypassed, appeared to be a powerful tool in the war against drugs.

As previously mentioned, urinalysis can be used to identify drug users but cannot measure impairment or the level of deteriorated performance. As well, it cannot distinguish recreational or casual users of drugs from those who are experiencing habituation, dependence, or drug-abuse problems. This form of testing can only be used to determine whether drug metabolites are present in the urine; it cannot determine whether these metabolites are active or inert. Since different drugs are eliminated from the body at different rates, drug tests can detect the use of some drugs more readily than others. For example, cannabis can be detected if it was used as long ago as three weeks prior to the test, whereas cocaine can only be detected if it was used within a few days (Kapur, 1994).

In addition to the United States government's goal of reducing drugs in society, another frequently stated aim of drug testing is to reduce the likelihood of industrial accidents. Policy statements from various countries including Canada, Australia, France, Sweden, and the Netherlands reveal, either implicitly or explicitly, that safety is the only reasonable justification for workplace drug-testing programs (International Labour Organization, 1994). The United States has indicated that the same regulations it has implemented for transportation employees, rationalized on the basis of safety, should also apply to other countries whose employees transport goods into the United States (McInally, 1995). As well, American subsidiaries that operate in Canada have been pressured to implement drug testing.

In Canada, drug testing has been less common than in the US and concentrated among companies in the transportation sector. In Ontario, about 4 percent of worksites had drug-testing programs in 1993, compared to 10 percent in 1989 (Macdonald & Wells, 1994). Another study of federally regulated transportation companies across Canada indicated 19.5 percent had drug testing in 1991 (Macdonald & Dooley, 1991). Recent unpublished data, from a 2003 survey of Canadian worksites with 100 or more employees, shows about 14 percent have drug testing, though in the transportation, communications, and utilities sector this jumps to 43 percent. Larger Canadian companies are also more likely to have drug-testing programs than smaller ones.

The Canadian Perspective on Drug Testing

Canadian culture has not embraced drug testing with the same enthusiasm as has the United States. In 1990, Transport Canada developed a strategy document for mandatory drug testing in safety-sensitive positions that also highlighted increased education and enhanced Employee Assistance Programs (EAPs) as important components of substance-use prevention. The plan received much opposition through a public consultation process, and the government aborted its attempt to introduce mandatory drug testing. According to McInally (1995), much of the opposition to drug testing stems from the inaccuracy of urinalysis to detect drug impairment. Since drug tests cannot detect impairment, opponents argue that they cannot be very effective at identifying whether employees are fit for work. A related and critical question is whether employers need an indirect tool to assess work performance, or whether they should rely on direct observations to see if employees are meeting the work criteria for their positions.

Legal challenges to the drug testing of employees have been based on violations of the Canadian Charter of Rights and Freedoms, Human Rights Legislation, and under collective bargaining or labour arbitration (McInally, 1995). The legality of drug testing has been challenged in the Canadian courts; and although no judgements have been made in the Supreme Court, several employers have been ordered to revise various aspects of their drug-testing policies. In the well-publicized case of Entrop v. Imperial Oil

Ltd, both pre-employment and random drug testing were determined to be violations of human-rights laws because they cannot assess actual or future impairment on the job.

In Canada, most employers who conduct drug testing for employees are in the safety-sensitive sector (Macdonald & Wells, 1994). The US goal of drug testing to reduce drug use in society as a whole or to reduce performance problems not related to safety, such as absenteeism, have generally not been acceptable reasons for drug testing in Canadian culture. During the late 1980s and early 1990s, many Canadian organizations developed policy papers on the value of drug testing in the workplace. Organizations that developed policy papers on drug testing include the following: addiction agencies such as the Addiction Research Foundation (1993) and the Alberta Alcohol Drug Abuse Commission (2000); legal groups including the Ontario Law Reform Commission (1992); unions led by the Canadian Labour Council (1986) and the Ontario Federation of Labour (1992); and human-rights groups including the Privacy Commission (1990) and the Canadian Human Rights Commission (2004). All these groups recommended against drug testing or suggested drug testing might be used under limited conditions (Table 4.1).

Given the wide endorsement of drug testing by governments and businesses in the United States, an intriguing question remains: why is drug testing so much less acceptable and desirable in Canada? One fundamental difference between the two nations is that in Canada, the only legally defensible reason for testing is to improve safety in the workplace; whereas in the United States, a key aim of drug testing is to reduce drug use in society. Clear cultural differences exist between the two countries in how each addresses issues of substance use. In the United States the emphasis is on legal sanctions, enforcement, and punishment (MacCoun & Reuter, 2001), while in Canada, more emphasis is placed on treatment and prevention of substance abuse, which is closer in intent to the goal of producing wellness. Drug testing is an enforcement/punitive approach, which is more in line with the American philosophy of a "War on Drugs" to deal with substance-use problems. Also, American laws permit greater employer powers than exist in Canada, which has a stronger labour and social-justice history.

Given that the only justification for drug testing in Canada is to improve workplace safety, a review of research in this field is worthwhile. Two questions are relevant. First, what is the research evidence that drugs are a substantial cause of work injuries? Second, what is the effectiveness of drug testing for reducing workplace accidents?

Table 4.1: Summary of policy recommendations
from major Canadian organizations

Type of organization	Name	Date of policy	Summary of major recommendation
Substance abuse	Addiction Research Foundation (ARF)	1993	• Does not recommend mass or random drug testing. • Reasonable-grounds testing could be considered for safety-sensitive positions. • Alcohol testing justifiable in safety-sensitive positions.
Substance abuse	Alberta Alcohol and Drug Abuse Commission (AADAC)	1988 (revised 2000)	• Does not recommend alcohol and drug testing except where substance use is affecting job performance. • If testing is used, it should be part of a broader company policy on substance use.
Legal reform	Ontario Law Reform Commission	1992	• A ban should exist on all drug and alcohol testing • Performance testing that evaluates psychomotor skills is justifiable in safety-sensitive positions.
Union	Canadian Labour Congress	1986	• Opposed to mandatory drug testing, voluntary testing, and employment-related drug screening for job applicants. • Preventive education and treatment centres should be expanded.
Union	Ontario Federation of Labour	1992	• Any form of employment-related drug or alcohol testing should be prohibited. • Prevention, education, and rehabilitation for alcohol and drug use should be expanded.

(cont.)

			• Joint union/management employee assistance programs should be expanded.
Human rights	Ontario Human Rights Commission	1996	• Drug testing cannot be justified for non-safety-sensitive positions, but may be permissible for safety-sensitive positions provided there is no other feasible method to ensure employees are not incapacitated on the job. • All positive tests must be accommodated and employees who are not substance-dependent must be returned to work.
Human rights	The Privacy Commissioner of Canada	1990	Random mandatory drug testing may be justifiable if • there are reasonable grounds to believe there is significant impairment within the group • drug use poses a substantial threat to safety • behaviour of group members cannot otherwise be supervised • drug testing can significantly reduce the risk to safety • no less intrusive alternatives would significantly reduce the risk to safety.
Human rights	Canadian Human Rights Commission	2004	• Pre-employment and random drug testing are unacceptable.

(cont.)

		• Random alcohol testing is permissible in safety-sensitive positions.
		• reasonable-cause or post-accident testing is acceptable if there are reasonable grounds to believe there is an underlying substance-abuse problem or impairment on the job.
		• Periodic or random testing following disclosure of alcohol/drug abuse or dependency may be acceptable.

Substance use as a cause of workplace accidents

Alcohol is the most commonly used drug in Canada with approximately 72.3 percent of the population drinking (Health Canada, 1995), and it is also the most frequently used psychoactive substance on the job (Stallones & Kraus, 1993). Use of other types of drugs is far less common. In Canada, survey respondents reported the following drug use in the 12 months prior to the study: sleeping pills (8.2 percent), marijuana/hashish (7.4 percent), tranquilizers (4.3 percent), stimulants (0.9 percent), and cocaine (0.7 percent) (Health Canada, 1995). Evidence concerning the prevalence of substance use on the job is sparse; however, most surveys generally indicate that less than 10 percent of respondents who use drugs also report using drugs at the workplace on at least one occasion during various periods of time (Newcomb, 1994). Therefore, drug use does not appear to be very common in the workplace.

The psychopharmacological properties of drugs assessed through laboratory studies are also relevant in assessing whether drug use might be a cause of job accidents. All studies indicate that the acute effects of alcohol impair psychomotor skills. For other drugs, research has shown that deficits in psychomotor co-ordination vary considerably, depending on the drug. For example, most laboratory studies have *not* shown cocaine to produce significant performance deficits. Although the evidence is more mixed for cannabis, alcohol is clearly related to poorer performance (Coambs & McAndrews, 1994). As well, the addictive effects, and those which cause harm in the long term, vary considerably among the drug classes. For example, compared to cannabis, cocaine is more problematic and more likely to interfere with an individual's employability.

Epidemiological studies are also useful for determining whether drug use is a substantial cause of workplace accidents. Some studies suggest that drug users as a group may have higher rates of job accidents than non-users (Macdonald, 1997). Other studies have failed to detect significant differences between drug users and non-users, and virtually all epidemiological studies have failed to show that drug use causes workplace accidents. With the exception of studies that focus exclusively on alcohol, there is no research that shows whether those involved in on-the-job accidents were actually under the influence of a drug at the time of their accident. Little research evidence exists to indicate the negative effects of different drugs on work performance. There is considerably more evidence that alcohol use at work may increase the likelihood of job accidents, with estimates ranging from 3 percent to 11 percent (Stallones & Kraus, 1993; Webb et al., 1994). Overall, research evidence suggests that alcohol is the drug that produces the greatest safety risk in the workplace (Single, 1998).

Drug users, as a group, may possess other characteristics, such as a propensity to take risks, which may be a more important cause of job accidents than the use of drugs. However, a wide range of factors contribute to workplace accidents. The most important of these stem from the condition of the workplace itself, such as inadequate work procedures, poorly maintained equipment, and inadequate training and supervision. Sleep problems and shift work were found to be more important contributors to workplace accidents than drug use (Macdonald, 1995). Overall, the research evidence suggests that drug use is *not* a major contributor to job accidents. This conclusion is drawn from studies on the prevalence of drug use, laboratory studies on the effects of drugs, and epidemiological research.

The effectiveness of drug testing for reducing workplace accidents

The effectiveness of drug testing for reducing job accidents can be measured empirically with outcome studies; however, little of this type of research has been conducted. Of the few studies that have been conducted, the evidence is inconclusive. Some authors have indicated that drug testing should be an effective means of reducing drug use by drawing on deterrence theory.[1] In fact, some studies have found that the percent of employees who test positive declined significantly after a testing program has been implemented (Macdonald & Wells, 1994).

In a recent review of evaluation studies of injuries, Kraus (2001) concluded that shortcomings in study designs and limitations of data preclude conclusions regarding the effectiveness of drug testing in reducing job accidents. In one study, job accidents were documented before and after the introduction of workplace drug testing (Taggart, 1989). Reductions in job accidents were found subsequent to drug testing; however, this study has been severely criticized for methodological problems because major safety improvements occurred at the same time that testing was initiated and no control group was used, making conclusions unreliable (Jones, 1990). A common practice of employers is to fire employees who test positive for drugs. Interestingly, no evaluation study has been located in the literature on the performance of such employees prior to their dismissal compared to matched control subjects. One conclusion that can be drawn from existing research is that there is no credible research evidence that drug testing programs will reduce job accidents.

Criteria for Assessing the Justifiability of Drug Testing in the Canadian Workplace

Assessing the justification for drug testing in the workplace may be based on weighing the benefits against the drawbacks. Employees' rights and duties must be balanced against those of employers. The nature of rights and duties for employers and employees is addressed by our legal systems, which are also partially a reflection of our societal values. As previously discussed, drug testing raises many scientific questions that can be useful for an examination of the rights of the employer versus those of the employee.

Employer rights and duties

Legislation governing employer rights and duties varies by province in Canada. The case in favour of drug testing is based on employers' rights to ensure certain job standards for employees and a duty to ensure certain work conditions, such as a safe workplace.

Employee rights and duties

Generally, employees have the right to be informed of potential hazardous working conditions and to be trained about safe working conditions. Workers also have a duty to work safely. Employees have other general rights as well, such as privacy, security, equality, and dignity. In some provinces, such as Ontario, employees have the right to be part of the process of identifying and resolving workplace health and safety concerns through participation on joint health and safety committees.

The balancing of employer and employee rights and duties
In order to assess whether drug testing is justified, we must consider
employer rights and duties against those of the employee. Clearly, as can
be seen from Table 4.1, Canadian organizations that have drafted policy
recommendations on drug testing have favoured employee rights over
those of the employer, as no policy was found where drug testing was fully
endorsed. There are several reasons that policies do not favour drug testing.
First, since drug tests do not measure impairment on the job (Kapur, 1994),
drug testing has been severely criticized because there is little correlation
between the test results and the employee's ability to perform on the job
(Borovoy, 1990). The exception to this rule is alcohol, where breathalysers
are typically used, and the test results correlate closely with actual levels
of impairment. The research evidence indicates that only a small percent
of people who use drugs use them during working hours. Therefore,
the majority of those who test positive are penalized for their behaviour
outside of work. These individuals do not represent an increased safety risk
at work. In other words, drug tests are a poor measure of fitness for work,
and therefore do not even meet the test of employer duties to ensure a safe
work environment. In addition, drug testing discriminates against workers
who do not represent an increased safety risk.

As well, drug testing invades one's physical privacy. Drug testing usually
involves the analysis of urine, and therefore by definition, violates one's
physical privacy. Urine tests can also invade further privacy if a third party
observes the act (Oscapella, 1994). Another aspect of privacy relates to
how the test results are handled and to whom they are disclosed. According
to one expert on the issue of privacy, there is virtually no control over
how information generated by testing is used. This information is highly
sensitive and could be used for purposes unrelated to the primary issue,
such as pregnancy tests (Oscapella, 1994).

Finally, it should be noted that drug testing programs can be implemented
in several ways, and that some forms of drug testing are more harmful
than others. There are numerous types of drug-testing programs: pre-
employment testing, random testing, periodic testing, post-treatment testing,
post-accident testing, reasonable-grounds testing, and voluntary testing.
As well, there are different consequences for employees or job applicants
who test positive, from being denied employment to being dismissed, or to
being referred to assessment or treatment.

Drug-testing programs can be grouped into two categories: (i) testing
of specific subgroups where there is some suspicion that drugs might
be used, such as reasonable-grounds, post-treatment and post-accident
testing; or (ii) testing groups where there is no grounds to suspect drug

use by a particular employee, which includies pre-employment, random, periodic, and voluntary testing. Testing where some suspicion for drug use exists is less harmful than where no grounds exist, because testing is then justified on the basis of job performance. However, routine testing after job accidents is not warranted, unless there is some additional reason to believe a particular employee was under the influence of drugs at the time of the accident. Routine testing after job accidents has the potential to erroneously identify drug use as the cause of the accident. Drug testing when an employee has prior knowledge of when he/she will be tested is preferable to testing without any knowledge. Prior-knowledge testing such as periodic or voluntary testing is less harmful, as such tests are more likely to catch the subset of drug users who are truly addicted and unable to abstain before the test, and thus who are most likely to represent performance problems in the workplace (Macdonald, Shain, & Wells, 1998).

In terms of consequences for those individuals who do test positive, treatment is more appropriate than dismissal because employers have a duty to accommodate. Accommodation is a less drastic approach than dismissal. It is especially harmful to dismiss employees who remain fit to do the work for which they were hired; therefore, the use of both EAPs and disability-management programs is a preferred alternative.

Alternatives to drug testing

A less intrusive approach that has a greater wellness orientation and is less punitive than drug testing is Employee Assistance Programming, particularly those programs with a health-promotion focus (Shain, 1994). It is also theorized that healthy lifestyles will reduce the demand for psychoactive drugs. Education of employees on drugs and alcohol issues is another approach that may reduce use. Finally, more direct performance testing of reaction times and psychomotor coordination, as recommended by the Ontario Law Reform Commission (1992), is a more practical alternative.

Conclusion

This chapter has summarized research conclusions on the following topics: substance use as a cause of workplace accidents, the effectiveness of drug testing to reduce job accidents, and the drawbacks of drug testing in terms of employee rights. These conclusions are helpful for understanding why drug testing has not been recommended by Canadian agencies. Research has not shown a clear causal link between drug use and job accidents. As well, drug testing has not been demonstrated to be effective in reducing job accidents; moreover, the intervention itself is harmful in several respects.

In order to recommend drug testing, research must minimally

demonstrate that the benefits outweigh the drawbacks. Possible benefits of urinalysis testing in reducing job accidents remain unproven. They are not a good measure of fitness for work. Although some types of drug testing are less harmful than others, the benefits have not been demonstrated for any type. Drug testing should therefore not be advocated, and it is certainly no adequate means for creating workplace wellness.

Endnote

1. Deterrence theory suggests that people will refrain from engaging in certain behaviours if there is high probability of getting caught and the consequences of being caught are severe.

References

Addiction Research Foundation. (1993). *Workplace testing for drugs and alcohol: Where to draw the line. Best Advice.* Toronto: Addiction Research Foundation.

Alberta Alcohol and Drug Abuse Commission. (2000). *Position on employment-related alcohol and drug testing.* (Policy and position paper).

American Management Association. *A 2000 AMA Survey: Workplace testing: Summary of key findings.* New York: American Management Association.

Borovoy, A. (1990). *Letter to Max Yalden, Chief Commissioner.* Canadian Human Rights Commission, General Counsel, Toronto: Canadian Civil Liberties Association.

Canadian Human Rights Commission. (1988). *Policy 88-1. Drug Testing.* Ottawa: Canadian Human Rights Commission.

Canadian Labour Council. (1986). *Position paper on mandatory drug testing.* Toronto: Canadian Labour Congress.

Coambs, R.B., & McAndrews, M.P. (1994). The effects of psychoactive substances on workplace performance. In S. Macdonald and P. Roman (eds.), *Drug testing in the workplace.* New York: Plenum Press.

Executive order No. 12564, 51 Federal Regulation 32.889 (1986). Washington: Federal Government.

Health Canada. (1995). *Canada's alcohol and other drugs survey.* Minister of Supply and Services, Ottawa.

Health & Welfare Canada. (1988). *Canada's health promotion survey: Technical report.* Minister of Supply and Services Canada, Ottawa.

International Labour Organization. (1994). *Drug and alcohol testing in the workplace.* Geneva: International Labour Organization.

Jones, J.P. (1990). Drug testing did not reduce Southern Pacific's accident rate. *Forensic Urine Drug Testing,* 2–4.

Kapur, B. (1994). Drug-testing: Methods and interpretations of test results. In

S. Macdonald & P. Roman (eds.), *Drug-testing in the workplace*. New York: Plenum Press.

Kraus, J.F. (2001). The effects of certain drug-testing programs on injury reduction in the workplace: An evidence-based review. *International Journal of Occupational and Environmental Health* Apr–Jun 7(2), 103–8.

MacCoun, R.J. & Reuter, P. (2001). *Drug war heresies: Learning from other vices, times, and places*. New York: Cambridge University Press.

Macdonald, S. & Wells, S. (1994). The prevalence and characteristics of EAPs, health promotion and drug testing programs in Ontario. *Employee Assistance Quarterly* 10(1), 25–60.

Macdonald, S. (1997). Workplace alcohol and other drug testing: A review of the scientific evidence. *Drug and Alcohol Review* 16, 251–59.

Macdonald, S. (1995). The role of drugs in workplace injuries: Is drug testing appropriate? *Journal of Drug Issues* 15, 703–22.

Macdonald, S., & Dooley, S. (1991). The nature and extent of EAPs and drug screening programs in Canadian transportation companies. *Employee Assistance Quarterly* 6(4), 23–40.

Macdonald, S., Shain, M., & Wells, S. (1998). Assessing the justifiability of workplace interventions: The case of drug testing. *Canadian Labour and Employment Law Journal* 6(3): 369–385.

Macdonald, S., Wells, S., & Fry, R. (1993). The limitations of drug screening in the workplace. *International Labour Review* 132(1), 95–113.

McCunney, R.J. (1989). Drug testing: Technical complications of a complex social issue. *American Journal of Industrial Medicine* 15(5), 599–600.

McInally, L. (1995). *A moving target: A study of the development, evolution and demise of Transport Canada's strategy on substance use in safety-sensitive positions in Canadian transportation*. M.A. thesis in Criminology. Simon Fraser University.

Newcomb, M. (1994). The prevalence of alcohol and other drug use on the job: Cause for concern or irrational hysteria? *Journal of Drug Issues* 24, 403–16.

Ontario Human Rights Commission. (1996). *Policy on drug and alcohol testing*. Toronto: Ontario Human Rights Commission.

Oscapella, E. (1994). Drug testing and privacy: "Are you now, or have you ever been, a member of the Communist Party?" McCarthyism, early 1950s; "Are you now or have you ever been a user of illicit drugs?" Chemical McCarthyism, 1990s. *Canadian Law Journal* 2, 333.

Privacy Commission of Canada. (1990). *Drug testing and privacy*. Ottawa: Ministry of Supply and Services.

Shain, M. (1994). Alternatives to drug testing. In S. Macdonald & P. Roman (eds.) *Drug-testing in the Workplace*. New York: Plenum Press.

Simeon, R.E., Cherniak, E.A, McCamus, J.D., & Ross, M.A. (1996). *Report on drug and alcohol testing in the workplace*. Toronto: Ontario Law Reform Commission.

Single, E. (1998). *Substance abuse and the workplace in Canada.* Report prepared for Health Canada.

Stallones, L. & Kraus, J.F. (1993). The occurrence and epidemiologic features of alcohol-related occupation injuries. *Addiction* 88, 945–951.

Taggart R. (1989). Results of the drug testing program at Southern Pacific Railroad. In *Drugs in the Workplace: Research and evaluation data.* NIDA Research Monograph, No. 91. US Government Printing Office, Washington, DC.

The Privacy Commissioner of Canada. (1990). *Drug testing and privacy.* Ottawa: Ministry of Supply and Services, Canada (Cat. No. IP34-2/1990).

Transport Canada. (1990). *Strategy on substance use in safety-sensitive positions in Canadian transportation.* Ottawa: Transport Canada (Cat. No. TP10202).

Webb, G.R., Redman, S., Hennrikus, D.J., Kelman, G.R., Gibberd, R.W., & Sanson-Fisher, R.W. (1994). The relationships between high risk and problem drinking and the occurrence of work injuries and related absences. *Journal of Studies on Alcohol* 55, 434–436.

Wilson, G.F., Davis, J., & Signoretti, K. (1992). *The prohibition of employment-related drug and alcohol testing.* Ontario Federation of Labour (CLC).

Part II

STRUCTURE

5

Foundations for Program Development

Rick Csiernik

Introduction

As a human service located in the workplace, Employee Assistance Programming has a dual nature that needs to be addressed. EAPs serve both the needs of organizations and those of employees: they not only provide support and counsel to workers and their family members, but also assist in creating a productive and healthy work force. As such, each EAP needs to be uniquely designed for its workplace, taking into consideration the distinct requirements of both labour and management interests. This is typically accomplished through the auspices of a Joint Labour–Management EAP Committee, such as those found in organizations where employees are covered by a collective bargaining agreement. A fundamental element of the success of an EAP is the co-operation and commitment of both labour and management. Canadian Labour Congress Executive Vice-President Dick Martin states that:

> Unions have traditionally taken care of their own members not only by negotiating protection clauses in collective agreements, but they have always assisted members with problems which may or may not have arisen out of the workplace. A Joint (labour–management initiated) Employee Assistance Program is just another structure by which the Union can continue to struggle for the betterment of workers' and their families' lives at and away from the workplace. (Canadian Labour Congress, 1986: i)

Employee Assistance Programs have been demonstrated to be highly successful, both in human and cost-effective terms, benefiting employers, employees and the community at large (Csiernik, 1993; 1995; 1998; Houts,

73

1991; Mowry, 1996). They can be designed to accommodate small and large businesses, labour unions, professional associations, as well as both private- and public-sector employers. While EAPs are distinct to individual work-sites, they do share common characteristics and it is essential that every organization implementing or redesigning an EAP prepare a formal, structured plan for program development following a series of key steps. The process may take anywhere from three to twelve months, though some have taken much longer depending upon labour–management relations. Figure 5.1 illustrates a sample critical path for EAP development.

During this process there are several key questions to address for the program to move successfully from the theoretical to the applied.

Key Questions

The following issues must be given consideration when an organization plans to introduce an Employee Assistance Program, in order to help define the initial scope and nature of the program, and therefore outline its utilization and set goals for its effectiveness.

i)   Ownership: The Joint Labour–Management Committee
      Almost all EAPs are organized by some type of committee (Csiernik, 1997). The most common is the Joint Labour–Management Committee, with representation from various sectors/divisions of the company. Those who serve on the committee will add to the uniqueness that surrounds each work-site's EAP. However, care needs to be taken in committee selection to obtain the right blend of committed individuals who can attend meetings and who also represent the various factions within the organization. Both labour, unionized and non-unionized, and management should serve, as should any neutral parties such as the EAP coordinator or occupational-health nurse. The best format for leadership is to elect, not select, a chairperson once the committee is operational, although many new committees choose to begin operation using co-chairs, one from management and one from labour. Often once the EAP is operational, the EAP counsellor or co-ordinator becomes the chair. Another important consideration is the mechanism for committee renewal, so that the group does not become tired of the role or turn over too rapidly.
      Thus, the first question is: who will represent management and who will represent labour on the inaugural EAP committee charged with developing the program? Central to this is the question of how large the committee should be. Typically organizations choose to

Figure 5.1: Sample critical path

Phase

I   Management and labour agree to develop an EAP and form a joint committee

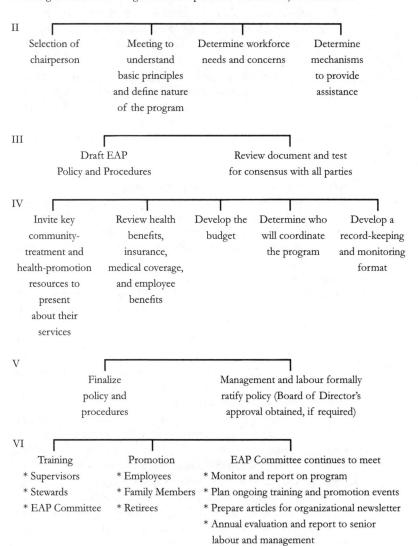

II

| Selection of chairperson | Meeting to understand basic principles and define nature of the program | Determine workforce needs and concerns | Determine mechanisms to provide assistance |

III

| Draft EAP Policy and Procedures | Review document and test for consensus with all parties |

IV

| Invite key community-treatment and health-promotion resources to present about their services | Review health benefits, insurance, medical coverage, and employee benefits | Develop the budget | Determine who will coordinate the program | Develop a record-keeping and monitoring format |

V

| Finalize policy and procedures | Management and labour formally ratify policy (Board of Director's approval obtained, if required) |

VI

| Training | Promotion | EAP Committee continues to meet |
* Supervisors   * Employees   * Monitor and report on program
* Stewards   * Family Members   * Plan ongoing training and promotion events
* EAP Committee   * Retirees   * Prepare articles for organizational newsletter
                                        * Annual evaluation and report to senior
                                          labour and management

provide a balance between management and labour representatives, with either human resources or senior management representing administration; and with members of the union executive, shop stewards, or union counsellors representing labour's interests. In organizations where there are non-unionized workers, they too can have a member on the joint committee. If the EAP opts for an internal model, the EAP coordinator should serve, while if an external provider is in place, a representative is typically expected to attend committee meetings, though in a non-voting capacity.[1] Likewise, if there is a medical department, the occupational-health nurse should be included, while many organizations also choose to have a member of the occupational health and safety committee represented in order to enhance communication with that related mandated committee.

While there is no best number of persons who should sit on the committee, size does limit the amount and quality of communication that can take place during a meeting. The greater the membership, the greater the number of interpersonal relationships that need to be managed. Six to eight is typically the most effective size for this type of small group, with its mix of process and task responsibilities (Toseland & Rivas, 2001).

ii) Availability and Eligibility

Once the committee is established, an early issue to address is who may actually use the program. Is the EAP intended for all sectors of the workplace, white collar, blue collar, pink collar, and executives alike? Can families use it, including partners of the same sex, making the scheme an Employee and Family Assistance Program (EFAP) rather than merely an Employee Assistance Program? What of probationers, contract employees, and retirees? If an employee is terminated or suspended pending discharge, may this person still use the program? Once decisions are made about who may use the program, the next question will often be how often an employee may use the program. Will the EAP allow persons with the same issue to use the program repeatedly; and if so, how many times is the organization willing to have an employee use the program in order to address a problem such as a recurring substance abuse? Likewise, can the program be used repeatedly if the employee has a range of issues that are causing him or her distress, and impacting work performance?

iii) Range of Services

Once it is known who will be eligible to use the program, it should be determined what types of services the program will provide.

Will the EAP be used primarily as an assessment or referral service, or will it provide counselling? Is the focus exclusively on alcohol and drug issues, or will it be a broadbrush program? Will the focus move beyond treatment and take on health-promotion and wellness-enhancing initiatives? Will a "rapid response critical incident debriefing" service or team, either peer or professional, be included in the program?

In helping to determine the range of services, the issue of who will cover the cost must also be addressed. Is the EAP an employee benefit, or will there be some co-payment by program users? In circumstances where management has not been receptive to working co-operatively to develop and implement an EAP, unions have organized their own labour-based and -managed programs, using union dues or a special levy to fund the initiative.

A final issue is when the program will be available. Will the EAP be accessible all day every day, or only during regular working hours; or perhaps a compromise with some weekend and evening hours of access? This choice will have an impact on use and of course on the total cost of running the service.

iv) Referral: Accessing the Program

Another question to be posed during the development of an EAP is how the employee, retiree, or family member will access the services. The preferable route is voluntary access, a method often predicated on health-promotion initiatives, as well as program outreach and promotion. However, the EAP committee also needs to consider the role and function of informal referrals to the program through the union, occupational-health services, and peers. Management often also wishes to include a formal component where employees, prior to or during the course of disciplinary action, will be asked to see the EAP counsellor to determine if it is a personal issue that is preventing them from meeting their job expectations. Each choice has implications on how the EAP will be viewed by employees, the types of problems presented, and at what point during the development of a given problem and individual will seek help from the service.

v) Program Promotion

Critical to the use of any new program is its promotion. Connected to the question of who is eligible to use the program is how the eligible employees will learn about it. The on-site workforce is generally a captive audience, which can be accessed through a variety of standard mechanisms, such as memos, staff meetings, flyers, posters, pay stuffers, brochures, telephone stickers, and even videos. However, how does the program wish to reach out to family members, retirees, and those who are not on the main worksite the majority of the time? While letters home, open houses, and refrigerator magnets are the standard fare for these groups, program promotion will need to be addressed and assessed both initially and on an ongoing basis.

In conjunction with EAP promotion is the training of staff. The EAP committee will need to consider who should receive special training about the EAP: supervisors, all management staff, and/ or union stewards. And should the EAP also use and thus train specialized referral agents? This choice will be closely linked with the referral options and access points to the program.

vi) Internal or External Program

The last question has created some of the greatest divisiveness in the EAP field: how will the program be delivered? Among the most

Table 5.1: Summary of internal EAP strengths and weaknesses

Strengths	Weaknesses
• use of an internal model will produce organizational cost savings • organizational belongingness and understanding of the dynamic environment of the workplace • higher utilization rates than external programs • organizational positioning and support • long-range perspective • immediacy of response to critical incidents • quicker response to organizational changes • knowledge of organizational policies and procedures • better positioned to respond to the Integrated Model of Occupational Assistance	• replication of resources available in the community • staffing may not be adequate to meet organizational diversity • ability for ongoing professional developmental opportunities • ethical conflict over who is the client and confidentiality perceptions • greater cost per employee

Adapted from: Christie, 1994; Csiernik, 1995b; Cunningham, 1994; Curran & Shirley, 1998; Favorini & Spitzer, 1993; Googins & Godfrey, 1987; Leong & Every, 1997; Ross, 1996.

Table 5.2: Summary of external EAP strengths and weaknesses

Strengths	Weaknesses
• use of an external model will produce organizational cost savings	• necessity of profit margin to maintain operations
• greater utilization by non-employees	• less awareness of organizational culture
• greater utilization by senior management/executives	• fewer informal contacts
• off-site locations promote feelings of confidentiality	• ethical conflict over who is the client
	• fewer supervisor consultations
• best option for smaller organizations	• slower response time to immediate crisis or critical incident
• wider range of clinical resources and greater likelihood to provide longer hours for access	• lower use of services for alcohol or other drug use and for work-related problems
• consistent service over broad geographic areas	• capped services
• provision of some service at a minimal cost	• fewer core services per employee
	• increased cost if threshold utilization rate surpassed
• more emphasis on and experience with marketing of services and self-promotion	• lack of consistency between intake and counselling services

Adapted from: Christie, 1994; Csiernik, 1995b; Cunningham, 1994; Curran & Shirley, 1998; Favorini & Spitzer, 1993; Googins & Godfrey, 1987; Leong & Every, 1997; Ross, 1996.

contentious issues in EAP is as follows: which is better, an internal program provided by one or more professional counsellors, either alone or in co-operation with specially trained peer-referral agents or union counsellors, or the services provided by a third party such as external private counsellor or counselling firm. Tables 5.1 and 5.2 summarize the key strengths and weaknesses of the two options of EAP service delivery.

In 1995 the results of the National Survey of Worksites and Employee Assistance Programs in the United States were released (French, Zarkin, Bray, & Hartwell, 1995). The study indicated that internal programs generally cost more per employee than did external programs, but that internal programs provided more comprehensive services than did their external counterparts (Table 5.3). Similarly, findings from Canadian Employee Assistance Programs have shown that internal programs have greater utilization rates and are more likely to deal with substance abuse and work-related problems. Those providing EAP services while also working for the organization itself typically have a better understanding of workplace dynamics and have a better organizational positioning than do external service providers (Csiernik, 1999).

Table 5.3: Internal versus external program costs in US$ (1995)

	Mean	Median
Internal (n=141)	$ 27.69	$ 18.04
External (n=478)	$ 22.19	$ 17.50
difference	$ 5.50	$ 0.54

Adapted from: French, Zarkin, Bray & Hartwell, 1995b.

Of course the ultimate solution would be to implement a combined internal–external program. This could utilize a mix of resources including referral agents, union counsellors, self-help groups, an EAP coordinator, and short-term counselling specialists integrated with external providers who work with long-term or very specific issues such as violence and trauma, compulsive behaviours, or identified substance abusers. Disadvantages inherent in both internal and external models can be minimized by using a dual pathway, and thus finding common ground between the two prominent factions within the EAP profession.

Conclusion

The answers to the above questions will affect the nature of the EAP, particularly in terms of the kind of assistance provided and to whom, and this will ultimately have a significant effect on worker and organization wellness. Where feasible, the ultimate solution for organizations committed to providing the best possible EAP service would be to use a Joint Labour–

Management Committee to ensure that a formal plan is developed and evaluated which involves all key stakeholders. Furthermore, once the program is established, the EAP or EFAP Committee should be charged with continuing to pose questions about the ongoing growth, development, and evolution of the program.

Endnotes
1. See Chapter 6.

References

Canadian Labour Congress. (1986). *Joint Employee Assistance Programme*. Ottawa: Canadian Labour Congress.

Christie, J. (1994). Grazing in each other's pastures: Internal and external EAPs. *EAPA Exchange* 24(6), 18–19.

Csiernik, R. (1993). The value of Employee Assistance Programming. *Canadian Review of Social Policy* 32, 68–73.

Csiernik, R. (1995a). A review of research methods used to examine Employee Assistance Program delivery options. *Evaluation and Program Planning* 18 (1), 25–36.

Csiernik, R. (1995b). *Developing an Employee Assistance Program: Essential aspects and components*. Hamilton: McMaster University.

Csiernik, R. (1997). The relationship between program developers and the delivery of occupational assistance. *Employee Assistance Quarterly* 13 (2), 31–53.

Csiernik, R. (1998). A profile of Canadian Employee Assistance Programs. *Employee Assistance Research Supplement* 2 (1), 1–8.

Csiernik, R. (1999). Internal versus external Employee Assistance Programs: What the Canadian data adds to the debate. *Employee Assistance Quarterly* 15 (2), 1–12.

Cunningham, G. (1994). *Effective Employee Assistance Programs*. Thousand Oaks: Sage.

Curran, J. & Shirley, J. (1998). An internal EAP: The best fit for Philadelphia Newspapers., *EAPA Exchange* 28(4), 35.

Favorini, A. & Spitzer, K. (1993). The emergence of External Employee Assistance Programs: Report of a survey and identification of trends. *Journal of Employee Assistance Research*, 2(1), 23–35.

French, M., Zarkin, G., Bray, J., & Hartwell, T. (1995). *Costs of Employee Assistance Programs: Comparison of national estimates from 1993 and 1995*. Rockville: National Institute on Drug Abuse.

French, M., Zarkin, G., Bray, J. & Hartwell, T. (1995b). Internal versus external program costs in United States dollars. (1995). *Journal of Behavioral Health Services and Research*, 26(1), 95-103.

Googins, B. & Godfrey, J. (1987). *Occupational social work*. Toronto: Prentice-Hall.

Houts, L. (1991). Survey of the current status of cost-savings evaluations in Employee Assistance Programs. *Employee Assistance Quarterly* 7(1), 57–72.

Leong, D. & Every, D. (1997) Internal and external EAPs: Is one better than the other? *Employee Assistance Quarterly* 12(3), 47–62.

Mowry, S. (1996*). Prince Edward Island Public Sector Employee Assistance Program Evaluation*. Charlottetown: Government of Prince Edward Island.

Ross, G. (1996). Marketing internal Employee Assistance Programs: What brings them in? *EAPA Exchange* 26(1), 26–27.

Toseland, R. & Rivas, R. (1997). *An introduction to group work practice* (3rd edn). Needham Heights: Allyn & Bacon.

6

Governance:
Best Practices in Policy Development

Rick Csiernik

Introduction

Best practices are those actions that have the greatest impact on enhancing the delivery of services to the targeted population. They include principles, guidelines, resources, research, the actual programs, and the policies that guide the programs. These actions should be not only the most effective, but also the most appropriate for a specific situation based upon available knowledge and capacities. Best-practices action thus necessitates the synthesis and consolidation of both empirical knowledge and practice wisdom (Manske & Maule, 2001). In theory, the goal of each organization's Employee Assistance Program should be specified in a policy created prior to the implementation of the program and then regularly reviewed and updated.

An examination of EAP development identified eight specific stages in the development of the majority of successful EAPs. These stages begin with stimulating organizational interest in developing a program (Albert & Macdonald, 1982). This was followed by preliminary program planning, obtaining organizational commitment, creating a formal committee, preliminary policy development, formalization of the policy followed by institutionalizing the policy, which entailed the assignment of resources to allow the program to be implemented. The eighth and final phase entailed the actual implementation of the policy, which implied that the EAP had become functional and was being used by employees. The goal of this process was to institutionalize formally the Employee Assistance Program within the organization's culture, while maximizing the participation of both management and labour groups. It has been demonstrated that organizations that have implemented a policy tend to have a greater concern for worker welfare (Putname & Stout, 1985), and that EAP policies are valuable in protecting employees' rights (Soto, 1991). They also promote earlier program use through enhancing voluntary referrals and protecting confidentiality (Macdonald & Dooley, 1990).

However, organizations were found to be hesitant to introduce a policy when leaders believed its adoption and implementation would hinder the reputation of the organization, potentially indicating some type of internal organizational problem, or when an EAP would usurp existing internal employee control protocols (Putname & Stout, 1985). While a literature exists discussing the value, importance, and utility of having an EAP policy,[1] there have been few guidelines on what type of information should be contained within an actual policy.

Best-Practice Guidelines

While EAPs are unique to each individual workplace, there are common characteristics that should enhance their success. It is not only valuable but also prudent for an organization to prepare a formal, written policy outlining the intent of the program. The statement should contain an introductory descriptive statement, define responsibilities of key work-site persons, and discuss procedural issues. A policy also gains in status when it is signed and endorsed by both senior management and labour officials. The following items are suggestions for creating best-practice guidelines when developing, reviewing, or revising an EAP policy statement.

    i)   Principals and Intent of the Program:

        The purpose of our EAP is to help all employees, and their family members, who may develop social, behavioural, work, or health problems that could affect their work performance, their health and safety, or the productivity of the workplace. Our EAP will provide assistance to all employees, retirees, and members of their immediate family in obtaining an assessment, counselling, or appropriate referral and treatment for personal or work-related problems. Our EAP is restorative and preventative; it is not punitive in nature or intent.

        The introductory paragraph of an EAP policy should include an opening statement with a philosophy similar to the above example, along with statements discussing the following:

        a)   any additional reasons why the organization and affiliated labour groups endorse the Employee Assistance Program;

        b)   that the employer's interest in employee problems are limited to their effects on absenteeism, job performance, and related issues surrounding productivity;

    c)   that any personal or family problem is responsive to counselling, treatment and rehabilitation, or improvement;

    d)   that the EAP is completely confidential. Rather than being held against an employee, a decision to use the EAP should be viewed as an indication of personal and professional responsibility;

    e)   that the EAP results in human and economic savings for both the employer and the employee; and,

    f)   that the existence of an EAP does not alter management's responsibility or authority. Neither does it alter union prerogatives.

ii) Management and Labour Endorsement

The written policy statement will ideally be signed by the Chief Executive Officer and senior labour leaders along with members of the EAP committee, and be presented conjointly to all employees as a joint, co-operative endeavor.

iii) Clear Procedures for Access

An EAP should facilitate easy access to services, providing anonymity where possible while always maintaining confidentiality. Access to the referral process should be such that confidentiality is preserved and undue attention avoided for voluntary, informal, and formal referrals. Any decision on the part of employees to seek help must not interfere with their position or employment.

    a)   Voluntary Use

    It has been recognized that those who voluntarily seek assistance for a problem are the most successful in resolving their difficulties. Training and educational procedures should be developed that both enable and motivate individuals to refer themselves for assessment to EAP staff, union counsellors, referral agents, or external resources. These procedures should also allow employees access to evaluation by professionals, referrals for counselling, treatment, and follow-up. Employers and labour groups are encouraged to emphasize voluntary use of the Employee Assistance Program.

    b)   Informal Referral

    An EAP policy should indicate the roles of labour, health services, peers, and management in the workplace in providing information about the EAP to colleagues who might benefit from the program, or in recommending that an individual or member of their family consider the merit of contacting the EAP.

c)   Formal Use

Each EAP should prepare written procedures for any action initiated by management, peers, health services, and/or labour representatives to ensure successful formal referrals for those unable or unwilling to benefit from voluntary or informal referral. These procedures should provide for assessment by EAP staff, union counsellors or referral agents; evaluation by professionals; referral for counselling or treatment; feedback to and from the referral source; and follow-up. Formal referrals should be based upon deteriorating job performance as noted by the immediate supervisor, and discussed when appropriate with a union steward.

d)   Follow-up

Individuals should have access to follow-up services to ensure they continue to receive the type of counselling or treatment support needed to successfully resolve their problems. Follow-up is a key component of any preventative program, particularly if counselling is limited by a service cap, as it assists in averting a relapse into a crisis situation where a person's health, wellness, or employment may again be threatened.

iv)   Confidentiality

The principle of confidentiality requires that no information of a personal nature be shared or discussed with anyone without the informed and written consent of the referred employee or family member. The EAP will not operate effectively, nor for any length of time, without clear guidelines and a strong commitment to confidentiality. Explicit written rules must be established specifying how records are to be maintained; for what length of time; who will have access to them; what information will be released to whom; under what conditions; and using what type of release form. The policy should also indicate how employee EAP records will be used for purposes of monitoring, research, evaluation, and internal and external reports. Client records kept for EAP statistical reports should never have names attached, and statistical reports should always be aggregate in nature so that no person or individual work unit can be recognized.

Any and all exemptions to confidentiality, such as legal requirements to report suspected child abuse or neglect or harm to oneself or another, should be clearly indicated in the policy and employees should be made aware of these exceptions prior to disclosing any information to the EAP service provider, volunteer or professional.

As well, the EAP policy should explicitly state that the workplace has no control over, nor can supersede the authority of, the courts of law to subpoena information pertinent to matters before them at any time. EAP records should never become part of an employee's personnel file. Work performance records prepared by management separate from the EAP can of course remain part of the employee's permanent personnel record. However, all records of participation in the EAP need to remain strictly confidential.

While anonymity is the ultimate goal of the EAP, confidentiality and anonymity are not the same. It is impossible to prevent co-workers from noticing that a fellow employee is not at work for an extended period of time, or is off at a particular time each week. Nonetheless, the reasons for the absence are not to be disclosed, keeping the nature of the problem situation confidential, if not wholly anonymous.

v) Joint Labour–Management Committee

Endorsement of the program, its ongoing maintenance, monitoring, and evaluation should be undertaken whenever feasible through a committee equally representing management, labour (both union and non-union), and interested third parties such as the external EAP service provider. As the committee's primary function is not directed toward individual assessment or counselling, a lack of clinical training should not act as a deterrent to membership. The essential qualifications for EAP committee members are an interest and concern in helping fellow employees and their family members, and a desire to obtain as much information as possible with respect to the operations of the program.

vi) Education and Promotion

a) Management, labour representatives, health, and other counselling staff should be thoroughly informed about their respective roles in facilitating usage of the EAP. Training for all groups should be undertaken and regularly updated.

b) It is important that employees, their families, and all others eligible for the program be informed about the organization's EAP and the services it offers, and be continually updated on new program initiatives. Information about the EAP should be made available to all new employees and their families, and be part of both the orientation process and the employees' handbook.

c) An organization should also make a commitment through the EAP to ongoing education dealing with prevention, health promotion, wellness, and the broad range of problems facing both individuals and their families.

d) The input of both labour and management should be sought when developing training programs. Distinct educational components for each group should be prepared and presented regularly.

vii) Communication

Communication should regularly occur between the EAP committee and senior management and labour, employees, the health and safety committee, the medical department, the disability-management program, the EAP provider, and EAP associations. Information updates about the program, within the confines of confidentiality, need to occur regularly to maintain the spotlight on the program and ensure its continued support and usage.

viii) Monitoring and Evaluation

a) The EAP should develop a record-keeping system that:

1. protects the identity of the client;
2. facilitates case management and follow-up;
3. provides ready access to statistical information;
4. indicates under-utilization by a specific sector or group; and,
5. can follow emerging trends or patterns in EAP need.

Monitoring can also assist in planning educational and promotional activities for the workplace.

b) Specific review periods should be established to examine the effectiveness of the policy and procedures and to provide an objective evaluation of operation and performance. The information can also be used to determine future program planning, education, and promotion.

ix) Insurance and Compensation Coverage

Those seeking assistance through an EAP should be eligible for the same medical and disability benefits as employees with other illnesses or issues. A review of benefits and insurance should be completed prior to an EAP's implementation, ensuring that plans adequately cover appropriate assessment, counselling, and treatment for a broad range of situations. These concerns include, but are not limited to, critical incident stress; alcohol and other drug use, misuse, and abuse; mental health issues; work-related problems; family and marital issues; or other personal concerns. All persons involved with the EAP should be familiar with provisions of the medical and disability benefit plans, so that they can advise employees and their family members clearly as to the extent, nature, and additional cost of any recommended counselling or treatment, and the available reimbursement.

x)   Roles

One final inclusion is the descriptions and definitions of the responsibilities of work-site participants involved with the EAP. These may be included in the policy document itself, or as an appendix. Any additional role-specific responsibilities arising out of the development of an EAP policy should also be added to an individual employee's job description. The following is an extensive list of roles and responsibilities, though not all positions will exist in every organization. In many workplaces some functions will not come into play such as a union counsellor or referral agent, while in other work-sites roles may be combined such as when an occupational-health nurse takes on the additional responsibilities of also becoming the EAP coordinator.

a)   Senior Management:

1.   Support the concept of EAP and work in conjunction with labour in program development.
2.   Endorse the written policy.
3.   Provide adequate staff time to plan and develop the program.
4.   Allocate financial resources to the EAP.
5.   Assign representative(s) to the EAP committee.
6.   Provide time for staff orientation to the program.
7.   Provide time for training and orientation for all managers, supervisors, and union officials.
8.   Ensure full job and benefit protection for any employee using the program.
9.   Request and respond to regular reports from the EAP committee.
10. Provide adequate sick leave provisions for persons presenting serious personal problems to the EAP.
11. Review and if required revise the employee benefits plan.

b)   Senior Labour:

1.   Support the concept of EAP and work in conjunction with management in developing a program.
2.   Formally endorse the written policy.
3.   Assign representative(s) to the EAP committee.

4. Morally and financially support members interested in becoming union counsellors/referrals agents.

5. Ensure job benefits and promotion opportunities are not affected by members' use of the program.

6. Encourage the membership to use the program voluntarily if they have personal problems.

7. Ensure that the confidential integrity of the program is maintained.

8. Assist in publicizing and promoting the program.

9. Ensure formal interviews are restricted to job performance concerns.

c) Joint Committee:

1. Ensure committee composition represents all sectors of the organization.

2. Define the mandate of the program and its procedures.

3. Write the policy statement, including descriptions of the responsibilities of key work-site participants.

4. Schedule regular committee meetings, typically no less than four per year.

5. Become informed about community resources determining the availability of facilities, the timeliness and cost of available counselling or treatment. Where facilities are unavailable, or there are lengthy delays for appointments, the joint committee should work within the community to upgrade the level of services, improve the timeliness of counselling, and ensure the affordability of assistance in a manner that makes it readily available to all.

6. Interpret program policies, responsibilities, and procedures to union, management, referral agents, social service agencies in the community, and others, as required.

7. Determine the structure of the EAP, including what type of services will be delivered to which groups, including family members and retirees, and how these services will be delivered.

8. Select an external service provider if required.

9. Obtain adequate resources to ensure the program's viability and success.

10. Prepare promotional materials and conduct orientation sessions for senior management and

labour, employees and family members highlighting the confidential nature of the EAP and the distinction between confidentiality and anonymity.

11. Develop or assist in the development of a training package for supervisors and union stewards.

12. Develop a monitoring system and evaluation process for the EAP in order to revise goals and make appropriate program changes as new needs dictate.

13. Maintain confidentiality and work for anonymity by monitoring all procedures, and if any breaches in confidentiality occur, ensure that they are immediately addressed.

14. Maintain open lines of communication and make regular reports to senior management, labour officials, employees, employee families, and community resources. Minimally, an annual report of EAP activity should be prepared.

15. Become involved in local, regional and national EAP groups and associations.

Note: Joint Labour–Management Committees exist in both unionized and non-unionized settings. In the latter, non-management persons play the same roles and can have the same impact on the program as their peers in unionized work-sites.

d) Program Coordinator:

1. Member of the EAP committee, typically as the committee chair.

2. Assists in policy, procedure and program development.

3. Assists in developing promotional and educational training for employees, labour, management, families, and referral agents.

4. Is familiar with and informs the EAP committee about community services.

5. Assesses and refers employees and family members as required.

6. Provides short-term counselling and case management to employees and family members.

7. Ensures follow-up of employees and family members who have sought assistance.

8. Provides general statistics about the program, ensuring confidentiality of all records and anonymity of clients.

       9.   Keeps the committee updated about the EAP's operation both orally and through written reports.

e) Referral Agent/Union Counsellor:

       1.   Understands the principles and concepts of the EAP policy and associated procedures.

       2.   Completes specified training, including knowledge of interviewing skills, community resources, and the organization's benefit package.

       3.   Acts as resource to the EAP and occupational health and safety committees as well as to any manager, steward, or employee who requests assistance.

       4.   Keeps apprised of relevant community agencies and organizations and shares information with fellow referral agents/union counsellors regarding the quality and timeliness of services offered by various groups and services, including waiting lists.

       5.   Encourages members to seek assistance when applicable.

       6.   Makes workers aware of the services of the EAP and what their rights are when they use the program.

       7.   Is available to colleagues and peers who wish to talk.

       8.   Appropriately refers peers and is available for follow-up support if necessary.

       9.   Ensures confidentiality at all times and anonymity when possible.

     10.   Explains the consequences to employees who decline assistance if the behaviours that lead to the EAP referral do not change.

     11.   Union counsellors have the additional responsibility of being accountable to the Unit Chief Steward and ensuring the Chief Steward is informed of all cases of employee discipline.

Note: The Canadian Labour Congress recommends a minimum of one union counsellor/referral agent per one hundred employees.

f) Supervisor:

       1.   Does not act as a diagnostician or counsellor; rather, limits intervention in an EAP context to discussing issues of employee performance.

       2.   Understands the principal concept of the EAP policy and associated procedures.

3. Establishes acceptable consistent performance standards for all employees.
4. Recognizes, documents, and monitors changes in employee work and behaviour patterns.
5. Consults with union counsellors, external service providers, referral agents, and/or occupational-health nurses, if unsure of what action to take.
6. Encourages employees and colleagues exhibiting performance deterioration to consider using the EAP voluntarily.
7. Helps employees identify job performance problems and provide suggestions for improvement. If a union exists and the employee requests representation, arranges for a union steward to be present at the meeting. Avoids any reference to specific problems.
8. Continues to monitor performance. If performance continues to decline, re-states the options an employee has, including using the EAP. Outlines possible consequences of continued job performance decline, including the process of the disciplinary protocol.
9. Ensures confidentiality throughout the process.

g) Union/Employee Representative (Steward):
1. Understands the principles and concept of the EAP policy and associated procedures.
2. Encourages employees who indicate that they have a problem to seek help through the organization's EAP program.
3. Explains that the EAP program offers confidential help and time off, if required, and explains disciplinary consequences to employees who decline help offered though the program.
4. Acts as an advisor when approached.
5. Ensures that employees' requests for help do not affect their job security and promotional opportunities. Also ensures that interviews are restricted to job performance concerns and that all records are kept strictly confidential.
6. Ensures that the rights of all members of the bargaining unit are explained to them at the time of referral.
7. Accompanies employees in formal interviews with management upon request and supports employees when an offer of EAP use is appropriately made.

8. Joins with supervisors in providing support and follow-up on the job.
9. Assists in EAP education and awareness to the membership.
10. Ensures confidentiality throughout the process and anonymity when possible.
11. Works in conjunction with union counsellors to ensure that both the wellness and rights of a fellow employee using EAP are protected.

h) Employee:
1. The employee is encouraged to seek assistance voluntarily, when necessary, for any behavioural or health problem.
2. The employee is responsible for maintaining or regaining satisfactory work performance.
3. When there is a problem detrimentally affecting work performance and appropriate counselling or treatment is obtained, the employee should continue with the negotiated counselling contract until its successful completion.
4. If an employee declines the help that is offered and his/her job performance and attendance do not improve, or continue to deteriorate, the employee may be subject to the standard disciplinary process as in the provisions of the collective agreement.
5. When an employee accepts assistance and/or counselling but after a reasonable period of time is still unable to bring work performance up to an acceptable level, the disciplinary process may still be applied.
6. Employees should respect the right to confidentiality of all fellow workers.
7. The employee is urged to forward concerns, suggestions, or recommendations about the EAP to the EAP committee or coordinator.
8. Employees should inform their family members about the purpose of the EAP and how family members can access the program voluntarily and anonymously.

i) Co-Workers:
1. Is aware that the EAP is designed to help employees and their family members, not to punish or terminate them.

2. Understands that covering up for fellow employees with personal problems only worsens the situation.

3. Attends all EAP orientation and training sessions.

4. Is supportive of any employee who is seeking assistance.

j) Medical Services:

When a Medical Services department exists it can play a key role in the EAP process. The involvement of physicians is advantageous, as they are able to make a diagnosis that is recognized as valid for insurance purposes. The occupational-health nurse, in the absence of a physician, becomes the medical liaison and can also operate as the liaison between the company, external EAP service provider, and Joint Labour–Management Committee.

Employees often present themselves to Medical Services when voluntarily seeking help for personal problems. Occupational physicians and occupational-health nurses are able to intervene positively when employees arrive with minor complaints which may be suggestive of other more serious behavioural or health problems. When applicable, the medical staff:

1. Appoints a representative to serve on the EAP committee.

2. Assesses, refers, and provides follow-up services to employees.

3. Familiarizes itself with the EAP policy statement and referral procedures.

4. Is aware of how the employee health and benefits plan applies to the EAP.

5. Works with other EAP personnel to encourage all employees to voluntarily participate in the EAP when necessary.

6. Maintains confidentiality and attempts to protect anonymity at all times.

7. Compiles a reference system of resources in the community.

8. Promotes health education and provides information on prevention and wellness to all employees and, where possible, also to family members.

9. Acts as a referral agent in arranging for outside services when necessary.

k)   Human Resources Department:
     It is frequently politically prudent to have the human
     resources department only peripherally involved with the
     EAP. However, in some organizations the human resources
     department needs to take on a more active involvement with
     the program. If this is not necessary, the EAP committee,
     coordinator, external consultant, or Medical Department may
     take responsibility for some or all of the following roles:
     1.   Serve a coordinating function between the employer,
          external service provider(s), and the EAP committee.
     2.   Interpret company disciplinary and supervisory
          procedures as they relate to the Employee Assistance
          Program.
     3.   Monitor absenteeism, accidents, unusual behaviour,
          and other job performance indicators.
     4.   Inform new employees and their family members
          about the EAP.
     5.   Circulate EAP information to employees and their
          families on a regular basis.
     6.   Keep apprised of EAP-related company benefits.
     7.   Keep management and union updated on all EAP
          modifications to which the committee agrees.
     8.   Coordinate and integrate human resources and EAP
          policies.
     9.   Provide performance-appraisal mechanisms to all
          supervisors to assist them in monitoring employee
          performance.

Application

While the existing literature in this area openly discusses the importance of
each EAP having a formal policy, little guidance on what should constitute a
policy has been presented. The proposals in this chapter have been applied
to create an EAP policy best-practices guideline (Figure 6.1). The guidelines
include five distinct sections: an introductory statement of principles,
procedures, program development, roles, and an overall document critique.
Each section is sub-divided to further allow each aspect of the EAP policy
to be separately appraised.

The *introductory statement of principles* tests for labour/management
endorsement, the range of issues the program covers, a discussion of job
protection, confidentiality and anonymity, and for a discussion of benefits
provision. Section two, *procedures*, reviews the three access routes for EAP,

Figure 6.1: EAP policy best-practices guidelines

	Maximum score	Policy score
1. INTRODUCTORY STATEMENT OF PRINCIPLES		
Labour and management support/endorsement	10	_____
Range of problems covered by EAP	10	_____
Job protection	10	_____
Confidentiality of program	10	_____
Anonymity of program	10	_____
Benefit provision	10	_____
Area 1 sub-total (maximum 60)	_____	_____
2. PROCEDURES		
Voluntary access to program	10	_____
Informal referrals to program	10	_____
Formal referrals to program	10	_____
Follow-up	10	_____
Monitoring	10	_____
Evaluation	10	_____
Area 2 sub-total (maximum 60)	_____	_____
3. PROGRAM DEVELOPMENT		
Training of supervisors/stewards	10	_____
Orientation of workforce	10	_____
Publicizing program to workforce	10	_____
Publicizing program to families/family orientation	10	_____
Community liaison	10	_____
(EAP groups, community services and related agencies)		
Area 3 Sub-total (maximum 50)	_____	_____

4. ROLES

EAP committee	10	_____
Management	10	_____
Labour	10	_____
Employees' group (non-unionized)	10	_____
Supervisors	10	_____
Stewards	10	_____
Employees	10	_____
EAP coordinator	10	_____
Referral agents/union counsellors	10	_____
Human resources (personnel/industrial relations)	10	_____
Medical department (OHN/occupational physician)	10	_____
Area 4 Sub-total (maximum 110)	_____	_____

5. OVERALL DOCUMENT CRITIQUE

Clarity	10	_____
Thoroughness	10	_____
Area 5 sub-total (maximum 20)	_____	_____

TOTAL (maximum 300)   _____   _____

PERCENTAGE SCORE:

(total score/300)

voluntary, informal, and formal, along with checking for the inclusion of follow-up procedures; program monitoring; and program evaluation. The *program development* section evaluates whether the EAP policy includes sections on training, orientation, and promotion of the EAP to employees as well as to family members, and whether there is any indication of liaison with EAP resources outside the workplace. The fourth section is a review of the various roles pertaining to EAP that can be found within a workplace, while the final section allows an appraiser to assess the clarity and thoroughness of the policy.

Each item in each section can also be individually rated; this allows for not only the presence or absence of a characteristic, but also its thoroughness. This best-practices guideline can be employed during the initial creation of an EAP policy, and it can also be used to assess and compare EAP policies, providing an analysis of policy strengths and limitations. In addition, it can be employed when an organization is reviewing and revising its program to assist in the ongoing quality-improvement process that is necessary when working with any type of dynamic enterprise.

Endnotes
1.   Battle, 1988; Dixon, 1988; Soto, 1991; Taylor, Holosko, Smith, & Feit, 1988; Csiernik, 2003.

References
Albert, W. & Macdonald, S. (1982). *Employee Assistance Program policy development in the division of regional programs.* Toronto: Addiction Research Foundation.

Battle, S. (1988). Issues to consider in planning Employee Assistance Program evaluations. *Employee Assistance Quarterly* 3 (3–4), 79–93.

Csiernik, R. (2003). A review of Canadian EAP policies. *Employee Assistance Quarterly* 18(3), 33–43.

Dixon, K. (1988). Employee Assistance Programs: A primer for buyer and seller. *Hospital and Community Psychiatry* 39(6), 623–627.

Macdonald, S. & Dooley, S. (1990). Employee Assistance Programs: Emerging trends. *Canadian Journal of Community Mental Health* 9(1), 97–105.

Manske, S. & Malue. C. (2001). A system for best practices. *Alberta Alcohol and Drug Abuse Commission Developments* 21(6), 1–3.

Soto, C. (1991). Employee Assistance Program liability and workplace privacy. *Journal of Business and Psychology* 5(4), 537–541.

Taylor, P., Holosko, M., Smith, B.W., & Feit, M. (1988). Paving the way for EAP evaluations: Implications for social work. *Employee Assistance Quarterly* 3(3–4), 69–77.

7

What Are We Doing?
The Nature and Structure of Canadian Employee Assistance Programming

Rick Csiernik

Introduction

> The EAP has been established to assist any employee, immediate family member or retiree in resolving a personal problem. The services provided will be professional, confidential, and available at the earliest sign of need. This program intends to make a positive contribution to the growth and development of each individual who utilizes its services as well as the company as a whole.
>
> Noranda Inc., Brunswick Smelter Division, Belledune, New Brunswick

As conspicuous as Employee Assistance Programs are on the Canadian landscape, the programs themselves remain surprisingly unexplored. While there has been extensive research conducted in the EAP field in Canada,[1] there has not been an extensive examination of the structure and functions of programs.

In response, a four-page survey was developed in 2001 in conjunction with a national advisory committee of labour, management, and service providers. Along with basic demographic information, the instrument asked when programs began, who initiated the EAP, who provided services, and what their qualifications were. Inquiry was made regarding referral routes, utilization, who was eligible to receive assistance, and for how long. Table 7.1 highlights the location of the respondents (7.1a) and their respective workforce sectors (7.1b). The greatest number of responses came from Ontario (40.3 percent) while Prince Edward Island had only one (0.7 percent) reply, as did the Northwest Territories. As well, 14 (9.1 percent) national organizations returned the survey. Government organizations constituted one quarter of the replies, followed by manufacturing (15.6 percent), health care (13.0 percent), and education (13.0 percent). It was interesting to note that 100 (64.9 percent) of the 154 responses came from the public sector. Workforce size ranged from seven to 60,000, with a mean of 3,144 and a median of 1,350 employees.

Program Development

> [the purpose of our EAP is] to provide a work environment that supports our employees' well-being
>
> Law enforcement, Ontario

Despite an extensive history of occupational assistance in Canada (Csiernik, 1992), the EAP field remains relatively new, as only 16 programs in the study were initiated prior to 1980. Nearly half of these (65 or 45.8 percent) were developed in the 1980s, while another 56 (39.4 percent) were begun in the 1990s. There still also appears to be ongoing growth as 21

Table 7.1: Organization demographics (n=154)

Table 7.1a: Location of organizations			Table 7.1b: Workforce sector		
Location	Frequency	%	Sector	Frequency	%
British Columbia	5	3.2	Government	40	26.0
Alberta	14	9.1	Manufacturing	24	15.6
Saskatchewan	9	5.8	Education	20	13.0
Manitoba	11	7.1	Health care	20	13.0
Ontario	62	40.3	Forestry	8	5.2
Quebec	3	1.9	Energy and utilities	7	4.5
New Brunswick	12	7.8	Law	7	4.5
Nova Scotia	9	5.8	Transportation	5	3.2
Prince Edward Island	1	0.7	Mining	4	2.6
Newfoundland	11	7.1	Sales and service	4	2.6
			Social services	4	2.6
Yukon Territory	2	1.3	Communication	3	1.9
Northwest Territory	1	0.7	Construction	2	1.3
			Corrections	2	1.3
National	14	9.1	Finance	2	1.3
			Food services	2	1.3

(13.6 percent) were created between 1997 and 2001 with five (3.5 percent) begun in the new century.

Table 7.2 examines who initiated the EAP. The majority of the workplaces in the sample (89.6 percent) were unionized, and this is reflected in program initiation, given that more than half of the EAPs were created by a joint labour–management group. Management and/or human resources were responsible for beginning nearly one third of the programs (31.1 percent), followed by labour (6.4 percent) and occupational health (5.8 percent). While occupational health services were extensively involved in Occupational Alcoholism Programs (Csiernik, 1992; 1997), this latter finding suggests that the health services are of decreasing importance in EAP program development. Also, smaller organizations were more likely to have had their EAP initiated by management, while larger organizations were most likely to have a joint labour–management group as the driving force behind program development.

Table 7.2: EFAP initiator (n=154)

Initiator	Frequency	%
Joint labour–management group	82	53.2
Management	48	31.2
Labour	10	6.5
Occupational health	9	5.8
Individual	3	1.9
Not reported	2	1.3

Service Delivery

[the purpose of the EAP] is the promotion of human wellness and the creation of healthier employees, families and communities.
Suncor Energy, Oil Sands Fort McMurray, Alberta

Table 7.3 presents the three primary sources of providing assistance through an EAP, and how much the survey respondents used each option. What was most surprising was not that the majority of programs (86.4 percent) used at least one professional counsellor outside of the workplace, but how many used a hybrid model. Nearly one third of the organizations (47) use a combination of internal volunteers (either referral agents, union counsellors, or members of a 12-step fellowship), in conjunction with an internal coordinator or counsellor, and at least one external professional counsellor. Another 30 (19.5 percent) organizations use an internal professional supported by a third-party external counsellor. Only six (3.9 percent) organizations in the study used internal volunteers alone to provide assistance. It was also interesting to note that while 133 companies do use external counsellors or counselling agencies, just over one quarter use external counselling as their sole mechanism for providing EAP services. As well, according to the survey, the larger the organization, the greater the likelihood that an internal professional will be involved in providing services to the workforce.

Table 7.3: Delivery of EFAP services (n=154)

	Frequency		%
	sub-total	total	
1. Internal volunteers		72	46.7
Referral agents	64		41.6
12-step members	15		9.7
Union counsellors	13		8.4
2. Internal professionals		91	59.1
Social workers	46		29.9
Occupational health	46		29.9
Human resources	35		22.7
3. External professionals		133	86.4
Multidisciplinary agency	86		55.8
Private practitioners	56		36.4
Assessment referral service	13		8.4
Consortium	7		4.5

Labour-initiated programs were the most likely to use internal volunteers to provide assistance (70.0 percent), followed by joint committee-initiated EAPS (56.1 percent) and by management-initiated programs (31.2 percent). The number of internal volunteers used ranged from 1 (n=4) to 300 (n=1) with a mean of 40 and a median of 15. The amount of education and training provided to internal volunteers varied widely. One organization provided its internal volunteers with only one half day of training, after which they were allowed to become part of the EAP, while another required three weeks of training. One (n=10) and two (n=6) weeks of training were not atypical, though nearly 40 percent of organizations using peer supports reported providing three days or less. Thirty-four organizations reported that their internal volunteers also received annual follow-up education and training lasting from one half day (n=1) to two weeks (n=3), with a mean of four days.

Those providing EAP services in Canada are a well-educated group (Table 7.4a). Nearly 80 percent of organizations use at least one counsellor with a Master's degree, while slightly more than 40 percent have at least one counsellor with a doctoral degree. As well, nearly 40 percent of EAP counsellors have a specialized diploma in Addiction Studies, while one third have EAP studies certificates. Of the 154 respondents, 119 (77.3 percent) have counsellors who were members of a professional association with

Table 7.4: Service-provider qualifications

Table 7.4a: Degree/diploma (n=139)

	Frequency	%
Community college	27	19.4
Undergraduate	33	23.7
Master's	111	79.9
Doctoral	56	40.3
Addiction certificate	55	39.6
EAP Studies certificate	47	33.8

Table 7.4b: Certification (n=119)

	Frequency	%
Registered social worker (R.S.W.)	76	63.9
Registered psychologist (C. Psych)	56	47.1
Certified alcohol and drug counsellor	46	38.7
Certified trauma specialist (CTS)	41	34.5
Certified Employee Assistance professional	33	27.7
Certified occupational-health nurse	22	18.9
Certified marital and family therapist (AAMFT)	9	7.8
Clinical counselling certificate	8	6.7

practice guidelines and ethical codes of conduct (Table 7.4b). Nearly two-thirds (n=76) of organizations use registered social workers to provide assistance through their EAP; this is followed by certified psychologists (n=56), certified alcohol and drug counsellors (n=46), certified trauma specialists (n=41), certified Employee Assistance Professionals (n=33), and certified occupational-health nurses (n=22).

Program Access

When workplace-based assistance evolved from Occupational Alcoholism Programs to Employee Assistance Programs, the emphasis remained on the employee. However, in the intervening years there has been acknowledgment that immediate family members should also be counselled through the auspices of these initiatives. This has been a contributing factor to a name change in many programs (from "Employee Assistance" to "Employee and Family Assistance"). In this survey, 144 of 154 (93.5 percent) organizations allowed family members to use the company program. There were several groups, however, that were not readily allowed access to the EAP by the organization: this included part-time employees (27.9 percent), probationers (42.9 percent), seasonal workers (44.8 percent), retirees (54.6 percent), and employees who had been laid off (63.0 percent).

Each of the 154 programs in the study allowed those entitled to use the EAP to do so voluntarily. Nearly three-quarters had an informal referral system in place with 74 (48.1 percent) encouraging peers to refer their colleagues to the program. Sixty-two organizations had a formal referral pathway to EAP as an option, while 49 (31.8 percent) also had a mandatory program usage component. However, only eight companies had drug testing as a method through which EAP was accessed, and all eight were private-sector organizations that used third-party providers for their service delivery.

The capping of service has always been a contentious issue in EAP. Four organizations did not respond when asked if their program had a maximum number of counselling sessions. Seventy-two (48.0 percent) did cap EAP use, while 78 (52.0 percent) did not (Table 7.5). Three (2.0 percent) organizations had a monetary cap, rather than a limit, on the actual number of sessions allowed. One organization allowed only two sessions, while two organizations allowed for three, and four organization allowed for four. In reality these are not EAPs or EFAPs, but rather assessment and referral services (and it is somewhat misleading to include them in the research). In each of these cases the average number of sessions was the cap. For organizations with a capped service from five to twelve sessions, the average number of counselling sessions was 5.1, while for the 78 non-capped organizations the average was 5.0. Simply stated, there was no difference in the average number of sessions between the two groups. Capping did not provide any real savings, and in fact where services were capped at eight, ten, or twelve, average use by employees and family members was greater than in instances where no formal cap was in place. This finding was not influenced by whether the organization was public or private sector, nor was it influenced by who initiated the program. EAPs that used internal volunteers were most likely not to have a capped number of counselling sessions (50 percent). Just under one third of programs using internal professional service providers did not have a cap in place, while 80.8 percent of programs with an external service provider did have a formal cap on service provision.

Table 7.5: Service capping (n=150)

Number of sessions allowed	Average number of sessions	Frequency	%
No limit	5.0	78	52.0
2	2.0	1	0.7
3	3.0	2	1.3
4	4.0	4	2.7
5	3.4	11	7.3
6	4.8	23	15.3
8	5.3	11	7.3
10	6.4	11	7.3
12	8.0	6	4.0
Financial cap	3.3	3	2.0

Program Maintenance

The EAP committee was at one time the foundation of Employee Assistance Programming (Albert, Boyle, & Ponee, 1984). In this survey 98 (63.6 percent) of EAPs were administered by a formally structured and sanctioned committee. However, the significance of this finding is that over one third of EAPs are not administered through any type of joint labour-management group. Seven (70.0 percent) of the ten EAPs initiated by labour had a committee, while 85.4 percent of those developed by a joint committee continued to be administered by one. Just over one third (n=17) of the management-initiated programs had an EAP committee, while only two (22.2 percent) of the nine of those developed by occupational health services had a committee in place to oversee and monitor the program and to nurture its development. The larger the organization, the greater the likelihood of having a committee, with size ranging from three to twenty-five members.

Two aspects that are required for an EAP to continue to develop, and to be used, are program promotion and supervisor training. However, one quarter of respondents stated that their program did not carry out any type of regular promotion; this was slightly more common for third-party providers (27.1 percent) than it was for programs using internal professionals (25.3 percent) or internal volunteers (20.8 percent). Twelve (7.8 percent) organizations stated that they conducted promotion campaigns as needed, while four (2.6 percent) did them infrequently. Just under one quarter of the organizations (n=35) held an annual campaign, while 19 (12.3 percent) ran quarterly campaigns, and ten (6.5 percent) had semi-annual promotion activities. While utilization rate is not necessarily a comprehensive indicator of the health of an EAP, utilization rate was nearly two percentage points greater for organizations that conducted promotion campaigns (9.6 percent) than for those that did not (7.8 percent). Similarly, 38 (24.7 percent) organizations reported not providing any type of new, employee orientation on the existence or function of the EAP. Those that provided an orientation for new employees had a program-utilization rate of 9.8 percent, compared to 7.2 percent for those organizations that did not (a difference of more than one third). Not surprisingly, the smaller the organization, the less promotion that was conducted (Table 7.6).

Sixty-two (40.3 percent) organizations did not provide any type of supervisor education or training regarding Employee Assistance Programming. Of these, as part of their service delivery (or their exclusive provider of assistance), all 62 used professionals external to the workplace. Only 36 (23.4 percent) of organizations had any type of regular training/ education program in place; another 27 (17.5 percent) stated that they conducted these as the need arose.

Program Components

> [we have] no policy or mission statement. EAP was added under [the] benefits plan with no formal program management of services.
>
>   Education sector, Alberta

When EAPs began to evolve, a "basic" program consisted of a policy, an orientation to the new program, and the provision of service. Since

Table 7.6: Program maintenance (n=154)

Frequency of activity	Program promotion		Supervisor training	
	Frequency	%	Frequency	%
monthly	5	3.2	0	0
bi-monthly	4	2.6	1	0.6
quarterly	19	12.3	6	3.9
semi-annually	10	6.5	4	2.6
annually	35	22.7	25	16.2
as needed	12	7.8	27	17.5
infrequently	4	2.6	4	2.6
never	43	27.9	62	40.3
not reported	22	14.3	25	16.2

then many extra features have been added. One hundred and twenty-two (79.8 percent) EAPs had a formal policy in place, which provided written documentation and the framework upon which the program was based. On the other hand, 50 (32.5 percent) had carried out some type of formal program evaluation. However, this meant that one in five EAPs in this survey had no policy statement and operated within the organization without a formalized mandate. Two thirds were unable to (or chose not to) provide some form of rudimentary evaluative information regarding their program. Fifty-eight (37.7 percent) EAPs also had a distinct substance-abuse policy in place in conjunction with or separate from the EAP policy, but only seven (4.5 percent) organizations had distinct drug-testing programs. Nearly half (48.7 percent) of the respondents had a disability-management program in place, while a greater number (61.0 percent) had established a wellness program.

The majority of organizations had a critical incident/trauma protocol in place (81.2 percent) with 41 (34.5 percent) having access to a certified trauma specialist as part of their service provision. Most organizations also provided counselling services throughout the day, seven days per week (70.8 percent). Interestingly, three-quarters (n=116) of the respondents also reported that their EAPs provided group training or counselling sessions on topics such as coping with organizational stress or change. Considering the origins of Occupational Alcoholism Programs and EAPs in the self-help movement, it was surprising to find that only 17 (11.0 percent) organizations provided access to mutual-aid/self-help groups on-site. Of these, seven had Alcoholics Anonymous or related 12-step groups that met at the workplace, one featured peer-led group debriefing sessions, and four promoted wellness-related groups which focused on topics such as nutrition or weight loss.

Utilization

Overall, the mean utilization rate across the 154 programs was 9.2 percent with a median of 8.4 percent, and a mode of 10.0 percent (n=13). Utilization ranged from 1.0 percent for an Alberta hospital and an Ontario forestry company to 30.0 percent at Dana Canada, an Ontario manufacturing company. There was slightly greater utilization among private-sector companies than public-sector organizations, and utilization of EAP services was greater in unionized settings than in non-union environments. As well, utilization was greater in organizations where representatives of labour continued to be involved in the program's maintenance and development through involvement in a Joint Labor–Management Committee. Utilization rates were also greater when volunteers were involved, when a formal policy existed, and when there was at least one promotion campaign a year highlighting the existence of the EAP.

The most important discovery, however, was that there is no uniform formula for determining utilization. Ten organizations did not calculate a utilization rate; six reported that they did not know how the utilization rate they were reporting was calculated; and fifteen relied exclusively on their external service provider. Of the 102 companies that did report a utilization rate, there were 19 different calculations used (Table 7.7). The most commonly used formula was new files per year by the number of employees (n=39). This was followed by family members plus employees using the EAP divided by the total number of employees (n=21), and then total number of employees using the EAP divided by total number of employees in the workforce, even though family members had access to the counselling and assistance offered by the program (n=14). In this latter case, family members were not factored into either the numerator or the denominator. Only one organization that counted family members using the EAP also considered the number of family members in the denominator; another organization calculated utilization rate by dividing new cases into the total number of households represented by the workforce. Four companies included not only family members and employees, but also retirees, though they divided this total only by the actual number of employees. One company that counted retirees in the numerator also factored them into the denominator to obtain their utilization calculation. Seven organizations determined utilization by dividing the number of referrals by the number of employees, and three used counselling sessions as the numerator. Other utilization calculations reported in the survey were based on individual and group counselling sessions, families per year, hours of counselling provided, number of visits, and new cases.

Three organizations, recognizing the complications involved in determining an accurate utilization rate, actually used two separate calculations. Of these three companies, two determined an employee-only

Table 7.7: How utilization rate is calculated (n=154)

19	no response
15	defined by service provider
10	not calculated
6	do not know
39	new files/employees (ongoing files not included)
21	family + employees/total employees
14	only employees using/employees (family can use)
7	number of referrals/employees
4	staff + families + retirees/employees
3	employees only/employees (no family service offered)
3	counselling sessions/employees
1	number of calls/employees
1	number of visits/employees
1	new clients + carry overs + families/employees
1	individual counselling + group sessions/employees
1	new cases/household
1	employee + families/employees + families
1	families per year/employees
1	employees + retirees/employees + retirees
1	hours of service provided
1	our utilization rate is actually a guess. I tend to focus more on costs

2 calculations

2	employee use/employee population	as well as
	employees + dependents/employee population	
1	number of people/employees	as well as
	number of contacts/employees	

utilization rate along with a utilization rate that considered use by family members. The third company was interested not only in use but also in the rate of contact. However, perhaps the most telling response was "our utilization rate is actually a guess. I tend to focus more on costs."

Further complicating this is the fact that there is also no common definition of how a case is defined, as illustrated in Table 7.8. Twenty companies stated that it was their service provider who defined what a case was; six companies stated that it varied. The most frequent reply (n=32) to this open-ended question was that one new case was defined as either one new individual client or as one new family. For 31 organizations a phone intake was equivalent to a visit and would trigger the opening of a case; by contrast, for 18 organizations a case necessitated an actual face-to-face counselling session. As well, one food sector organization in Alberta only considered a meeting as a case if some type of treatment plan was developed.

Table 7.8: How a case is defined (n=154)

20	defined by service provider
8	no response
6	varies
6	do not know
2	do not calculate
32	one new family or one individual = 1 case
31	phone call or visit
18	actual face-to-face counselling session
7	2 individuals = 2 cases, 5 family members = 5 cases
5	each new problem is a new case even if it is the same person
5	15-minute phone contact
3	family member counted with employee as one case
2	any contact that leads to referral
2	if client file closed and then client returns in the same year = new case
1	defined by area of service counselling versus group—1 client can be 2 cases
1	every 12 hours of counselling is a new case
1	45-minute phone contact
1	4 phone contacts or one visit
1	only a case once treatment plan developed
1	only new clients, any repeat client is not a new case
1	couple together = 1, couple apart =2

Different lengths of phone contact triggered a case for other organizations. For one company, at least 45 minutes of phone contact were needed to be considered a case; for another company, four phone calls were equivalent to one visit; five companies responded that a minimum of fifteen minutes of contact constituted a new case. Seven different organizations from across Canada stated that they determined a case by the number of people who presented for counselling. For each of these companies two individuals from the same family would count as two cases; if five family members were seen, it would constitute five distinct cases. In contrast to this, three companies simply viewed family members as extensions of employees and did not count them independently; one company stated that if a couple comes together it is one case, but if they are also seen apart it became two cases in determining the utilization rate.

Five organizations stated that if they assisted the same client with two different problems in one year, that it would constitute two cases. It is hypothesized that this is one mechanism used to overcome the restrictions of service caps. Another organization reported that after every twelve hours of counselling they considered the situation a new case; again, this could potentially be a creative way to circumvent capping of services for clients still in need of counselling. A third scenario, employed by two organizations, may also have arisen as a response to the capping of services. In these organizations, if a client's case was closed but the client returned at some later time in the same year, it was considered a "new" case and the client became eligible for a new block of counselling sessions. This could also be one response by counsellors to employment; for example, if they are not paid by the hour, but by the case. Thus, if more heads are counted, more counselling can be supplied to the client and the counsellor can claim remuneration from the third-party provider who is coordinating the provision of clinical services.

Utilization rates are regularly used to compare organizations' ability to assist employees. These rates are used in assessing what model of assistance should be used in certain situations; for example, if additional program promotion or development is required. Utilization is also used as a foundational evaluative tool. In quantitative research, knowing how to count is a rudimentary necessity. However, in the multi-million dollar, multidisciplinary, and unregulated field of EAP, which exists both nationally and globally, this fundamental concept is lacking.

Conclusion

HLC is concerned with the personal well-being of all employees and their families. It is recognized that a wide range of personal problems may have an adverse effect on an employee's well-being and ability to perform his/her duties. Personal problems can include illness (physical or mental), emotional problems, stress, financial, family, marital, legal, or other problems such as substance abuse. HLC's EFAP is designed to provide accessible, professional and confidential help to all employees and their family members who are experiencing personal problems through a process of assessment, short-term counselling, referral and follow-up.

Health Labrador Corporation, Goose Bay, Labrador

Employee Assistance Programming remains a growing enterprise in Canada; while third-party professionals are a prominent mechanism through which assistance is provided, peers and internal professionals also play key roles within many programs. Differences in EAPs arise depending upon who initiates the program, who provides the service, the size of the organization, and whether it is a unionized environment. There remain many areas that require continued program development, including policies, promotion, orientation, supervisory and peer education and training, and perhaps most importantly, work on developing uniform definitions of critical terms, such as what constitutes a "case" and how to calculate utilization.

Endnotes

1.   Csiernik, 1997; 1998; 2000; Loo & Watts, 1993; Macdonald & Dooley, 1990; 1991; Macdonald, Lothian, & Wells, 1997; Macdonald & Wells, 1994, MacDonald & Davidson, 2000; Massey & Csiernik, 1997; McKibbon, 1993a; 1993b; Newman, 1983; Rheaume, 1992; Rodriguez, & Borgen, 1998

References

Albert, W., Boyle, B., & Ponee, C. (1984). *EAP orientation.* Toronto: Addiction Research Foundation.

Csiernik, R. (1992). The evolution of Employee Assistance Programming in North America. *Canadian Social Work Review* 9 (2), 214–228.

Csiernik, R. (1997). The relationship between program developers and the delivery of occupational assistance. *Employee Assistance Quarterly* 13 (2), 31–53.

Csiernik, R. (1998). A profile of Canadian Employee Assistance Programs. *Employee Assistance Research Supplement* 2 (1), 1–8.

Csiernik, R. (2000). The state of the nation: EAP education in Canada. *Employee Assistance Quarterly* 15(3), 15–22.

Loo, R. & Watts, T. (1993). A survey of Employee Assistance Programs in medium and large Canadian organizations. *Employee Assistance Quarterly* 8(3), 65–71.

Macdonald, S. & Dooley, S. (1990). A survey of Employee Assistance Programs and health promotion programs at Ontario worksites. *Employee Assistance Quarterly* 6(1), 1–15.

Macdonald, S. & Dooley, S. (1991). The nature and extent of EAPs and drug screening programs in Canadian Transportation Companies. *Employee Assistance Quarterly* 6(4), 23–40.

Macdonald, S., Lothian, S., & Wells, S. (1997). Evaluation of an Employee Assistance Program at a transportation company. *Evaluation and Program Planning* 20(4), 495–505.

Macdonald, S. & Wells, S. (1994). The prevalence and characteristics of Employee Assistance, health promotion and drug testing programs in Ontario. *Employee Assistance Quarterly* 10(1), 1–15.

MacDonald, N. & Davidson, S. (2000). The wellness program for medical faculty at the University of Ottawa: A work in progress. *Canadian Medical Association Journal* 163(6), 735–738.

Massey, M. & Csiernik, R. (1997). Community development in EAP: The Employee Assistance Program Council of Hamilton-Wentworth. *Employee Assistance Quarterly* 12(3), 35–46.

McKibbon, D. (1993a). EAPs in Canada: A panacea without definition. *Employee Assistance Quarterly* 8(3), 11–29.

McKibbon, D. (1993b). Staffing characteristics of Canadian EAP professions. *Employee Assistance Quarterly*, 9 (1), 31–66.

Newman, P. (1983). Program evaluation as a reflection of program goals. In R. Thomlinson (ed.), *Perspectives on industrial social work*. Toronto: Family Services Canada.

Rheaume, J. (1992). Santé mentale au travail: L'approche des programmes d'aide aux employés. *Canadian Journal of Community Mental Health* 11(2), 91–107.

Rodriguez, J. & Borgen, W. (1998). Needs assessment: Western Canada's program administrators' perspectives on the role of EAPs in the workplace. *Employee Assistance Quarterly* 14(2), 11–29.

8

A Review of
EAP Evaluation in Canada

Rick Csiernik

Introduction

The Employee Assistance field is a multidisciplinary, multi-perspective arena of practice with a myriad of outlooks on how best to institute programming. Since the 1980s researchers have attempted to consolidate the limited, though important, research and evaluation findings from programs for the use of practitioners, EAP committee members, and human-resource leaders.[1] This chapter reviews formal Canadian EAP evaluations that have been published using Macdonald's (1986) five steps in a comprehensive evaluation:

i)   Needs Assessment: to determine overall program goals and direction;
ii) Program Development (case studies): to describe the program, its rationale and objectives;
iii) Input Evaluation: to determine if the program components have been correctly implemented;
iv) Outcome Evaluation: to determine if the program objectives have been achieved;
v)   Process Evaluation: to determine what the program is actually doing and how well.

Needs Assessment

An EAP should have, both at the time the program is established and on a periodic basis thereafter, a mechanism to assess the needs for employee assistance. The EAP needs assessment should be aimed at identifying worksite environmental, programmatic, personnel and stress related factors deleterious to employee well-being or productivity. Program decisions should be directly related to the assessment findings and be periodically evaluated in that context (US Department of Health and Human Services, 1986: 10).

In spite of the fact that most administrators are aware that EAPs need to be carefully planned according to the specific needs of each individual workplace, there was only one formal Canadian needs assessment found in the literature. However, Rodriguez and Borgen's (1998) survey of 90 EAP administrators in Western Canada did not pertain to program development, but rather to program enhancement. It was reported that the EAP administrators who were surveyed were aware of personal problems among the workforce; while employees and family members were using the EAP, there was still a need for additional training and program promotion to improve its usage.

Otherwise, no study regarding needs assessment in Canada was found in the literature.

Case Studies

The second step in the comprehensive evaluation process recommended by Macdonald is to describe a program, its rationale and its objectives, once it becomes functional. Case studies are exploratory yet empirical, descriptive and detailed studies using a range of research methods to report on and interpret a single example of a phenomenon (Merriam, 1988; Tesch, 1990; Yin, 1989). This type of evaluation has historically been the most popular and prominent mechanism through which the various forms of EAP have been discussed and described (Csiernik, 1995; 1997), and yet only six[1] case studies pertaining to Canadian EAPs were found (the most recent having been published in 1989) (Table 8.1).

The published case studies typically described large organizations, with an average workforce size of over 17,000, with half using internal sources of providing assistance and half using external. All the histories that were provided described the program's origins and outlined their EAP's policies and procedures. Two of these discussed the types of problems dealt with by the program, how employees were referred to the EAP, and specific case histories of a program participant. Excluding Bell Canada (one of the first EAPs to be developed in Canada), the average time between initiation and article publication for the remaining five case studies was 6.2 years, with a range of three to nine years. This is a sufficient time to watch a fledgling initiative take hold and develop significant effects on the lives of individuals and on the organization itself. This time frame is also more than adequate

Table 8.1: Case studies summary

Author	Year	Workplace	Workforce size	Program initiated	EAP delivery	History outlined	Problem profile	Referrals	Policies and procedures	Case history	Clients
Johnson et al	1989	Red Deer College, Alberta		1983	internal/external	Yes			Yes		154
Lindop	1975	Bell Canada	45,000	1951	internal	Yes			Yes	Yes	
	1975	Gulf Canada	11,000	1967	internal	Yes			Yes		
Lynch	1980	Interlock, Vancouver, BC	4,030	1977	external	Yes	Yes	Yes	Yes		141
Pergantes	1982	London, Ontario Consortium	14,000	1975	external	Yes			Yes		164
Van Halm	1988	MacMillan Bloedel, BC	15,000	1979	external	Yes	Yes	Yes	Yes	Yes	

Adapted from: Bennett, 1978; Burke, 1994; Chandler, Kroeker, Flynn & MacDonald, 1988; Groeneveld, Shain, Brayshaw & Heideman, 1984; Johnson, Docherty, Michalenko, Bucklee & Hazlett, 1989; Lindop, 1975; Lynch, 1980; Macdonald, Lothian & Wells, 1997; Mowry, Hogan, Moase, Montgomery & Harper, 1987; Ontario Addiction Research Foundation, 1990; Newman, 1983; Pergantes, 1982; Sargeant & Tepperman, 1987; Shain & Suurvali, 1997; Van Halm, 1998.

to allow for more extensive evaluation to supplement the primarily narrative case-study presentation.

Input Evaluation

No input evaluations were found in the literature pertaining to Canadian EAPs. This may be explained by a variety of factors including:

- the rudimentary nature of this type of evaluation;
- the lack of perceived value in the findings;
- that input evaluations are simply not routinely conducted; and/or,
- that the findings are not formally documented.

While this form of evaluation may not be or may not perceived to be of significance by program evaluators, it can still be of value for an EAP committee and an organization to investigate the desired intention of the program, and whether it is meeting those objectives.

Outcome Evaluations

An EAP should have a mechanism in place to evaluate the appropriateness, effectiveness, and efficiency of the delivery of services and program integration. Evaluations of the scope and appropriateness of client services, educational programs, supervisory training, and outreach activities should be performed on an annual basis and become part of the permanent program records (US Department of Health and Human Services, 1986, 16).

The most common form of outcome evaluation in the EAP sector has been the traditional cost–benefit study. This was true for the Canadian literature, with eight studies found (Table 8.2). The trend in EAP evaluation literature is for the majority of reports to be conducted by organizations which maintain internal programs, as additional cost and competitive factors have minimized research conducted by external service providers). In this instance all eight evaluations were of programs that provided EAP services using internal staff. However, as with case studies, there were few contemporary cost–benefit evaluations found, with three having been published in the 1970s, four in the 1980s, and the most recent in 1990. Despite this limitation, all the studies used multiple variables to assess cost–benefit. The most common costs studied in the eight reports were absenteeism (6), health claims (5), grievances (4), performance (3),

Table 8.2: Cost–benefit reports

Author	Bennett	Bennett	Bennett	Chandler et al
Year	1978	1978	1978	1988
Workplace	General Motors, Oshawa	Chevrolet Canada	Fisher Body Plant	Seagram Distillery Amherstburg, Ont.
EAP delivery	Internal	Internal	Internal	Internal
Method	pre-post client evaluation n=192	pre-post client evaluation	pre-post client evaluation n=95	self-report questionnaire Organization records n=86
Study time-frame	3 years	40 months	2 years	8 years
Variables examined:	absenteeism health claims sick benefits grievances WCB claims WCB costs	disciplinary action grievances accidents sick leave health claims	absenteeism health claims grievances accidents disciplinary action	absenteeism accidents disciplinary action grievances visits to medical personnel
Outcome	• decreases found in: lost time: 81.9% sick claims: 84.1% sick benefits: 80.0% WCB claims: 60.0%	• decreases found in: disciplinary action: 52% grievances: 49% accidents: 47% sick leave: 37% sick claims: 22%	• decreases found in: lost time: 41% sick benefits: 55% grievances: 52% accidents: 31% disciplinary actions: 51%	• absence rates halved four years post-EAP use • decrease in both accident and grievance rates

(cont.)

Outcome (cont.)	• No changes in: grievances, WCB costs			• majority of program users would recommend EAP to peers
Author	Groeneveld, et al	Newman	Ontario Addiction Research Foundation	Sargent & Tepperman
Year	1984	1983	1990	1987
Workplace	Canadian National Rail	Manitoba Telephone USWA Local 6166 St. Boniface Hospital Winnipeg, Manitoba	Ontario Organization	Central Ontario Grocers
EAP Delivery	Internal	Internal	Internal	Internal
Method	pre-post job performance of formal referrals	employee survey organizational records client survey	pre-post job performance n=116	pre-post job performance n=24
Study time-frame	2 years	1 year	2 years	18 months
Variables examined:	absenteeism lateness health claims performance co-worker conflict	absenteeism performance retention problem resolution	health claims sick days health benefits	absenteeism lateness performance
Outcome	• decreases found in: absenteeism: 45.9% lateness: 50.0%	• EAP use found to improve capacity to perform job and	• decreases found in: sick claims: 42.4% sick days: 21.0%	• Cost savings on three variables $47,500 with a

(cont.)

| Outcome (cont.) | health claims: 55.6%
work performance
issues: 65.8%
co-worker conflict:
76.9% | improved employee
situation
• absenteeism rate
decreased
• high level of trust of
program by users | sick benefits: 32.5% | 60% improvement in
performance
• EAP paid for itself
within one year of
implementation |

Adapted from: Bennett, 1978; Burke, 1994; Chandler, Kroeker, Flynn & MacDonald, 1988; Groeneveld, Shain, Brayshaw & Heideman, 1984; Johnson, Docherty, Michalenko, Bucklee & Hazlett, 1989; Lindop, 1975; Lynch, 1980; Macdonald, Lothian & Wells, 1997; Mowry, Hogan, Moase, Montgomery & Harper, 1987; Ontario Addiction Research Foundation, 1990; Newman, 1983; Pergantes, 1982; Sargeant & Tepperman, 1987; Shain & Suurvali, 1997; Van Halm, 1998.

and disciplinary action (3). The length of study ranged from one year at three Manitoba workplaces (Newman, 1983) to an eight-year retrospective analysis at a Seagram's Distillery in Amherstburg, Ontario (Chandler, et al, 1988). The mean was just under three years.

As expected with published EAP cost–benefit studies, each evaluation demonstrated significant positive financial implications for establishing and maintaining an EAP. Decreases in absenteeism post EAP use ranged from 41.0 percent to 81.9 percent, and decreases in sick claims were also in the 40 percent to 50 percent range (Bennett, 1978; Groenveld et al. 1984; Ontario Addiction Research Foundation, 1990). The reported savings for 24 program users over the course of six month at Central Ontario Grocers was $47,500, with a 60 percent reported improvement in performance (Sargeant & Tepperman, 1987).

Process Evaluations

Process evaluations are the most complex means of evaluating how EAP inputs translate into outcomes, and also how they assist in contextualizing the reported outcomes. Thus it is interesting to note that of the four Canadian EAP process evaluations found in the literature (two evaluations related to internal EAPs, one related to a consortium, and one related to an external provider of service) were all published in the 1990s, and represent the most current evaluation knowledge presented.

The process evaluations had a broad range of purposes (Table 8.3 on p. 126), including examining program use, effectiveness, satisfaction, and impact on the quality of life. Accordingly they employed a range of methodologies:

- employee, client, manager, and counsellor point-in-time surveys;
- key informant interviews;
- focus groups;
- document reviews; and,
- pre/post treatment questionnaires.

Again, the results largely demonstrated that the EAPs were operating as expected and providing benefits to the workplace, and thus to both employees and employers. However, process evaluations are also conducted to provide recommendations for future program development; this could be seen in suggestions that the EAP become even more pro-active (Mowry et al, 1997), and that the EAP focus even more on prevention and education than it currently did (Shain & Suuvali, 1997).

Conclusion

Is the glass half full or is it half empty? Nineteen published studies, one third of which were primarily descriptive in nature, and several others of which would not bear up to the scrutiny of an undergraduate research methodology course. There certainly is not an extensive Canadian EAP-evaluation legacy. Yet, in a field with great promise and much talk, but at best negligible support both academically and organizationally for research, 19 examinations of program design are still an accomplishment that is worth acknowledging. The practitioners and academic evaluators who did carry out needs assessment, describe program development, and examine what programs were actually doing, and then publish these findings, have enhanced the baseline of knowledge in the Canadian EAP field, a practice area that is grossly under-studied.

The evaluators demonstrated creativity and ingenuity through the range of methodologies and both qualitative and quantitative data-collection procedures employed. However, while this summary highlights the value of conducting research, it also further underscores the dearth of critical knowledge we have about EAP in Canada. Thus, perhaps rather than asking if the glass is half full or half empty, we should congratulate the evaluators on knowing that there is in fact a glass that needs to be filled, and we should all be encouraged to do so in the twenty-first century.

Endnotes

1. Csiernik, 1995; 1998; Jerrell & Righmyer, 1982; Kurtz, Googins, & Howard, 1984.

Notes

The two case studies presented in their entirety in Part IV were not included in this analysis.

References

Bennett, K. (1978). *Successful employee assistance programs*. Toronto: Addiction Research Foundation.

Burke, R. (1994). Utilization of Employees' Assistance Program in a public accounting firm: Some preliminary data. *Psychological Reports* 75, 264–266.

Chandler, R., Kroeker, B., Flynn, M., & MacDonald, D. (1988). Establishing and evaluating an industrial social work programme: The Seagram, Amherstburg experience. *Employee Assistance Quarterly* 3 (3–4), 243–253.

Csiernik, R. (1995). A review of research methods used to examine Employee Assistance Program delivery options. *Evaluation and Program Planning* 18(1), 25–36.

Table 8.3: Process evaluations

Author	Burke	Macdonald, et al.	Mowry, et al.	Shain & Suurvali
Year	1994	1997	1997	1997
Workplace	Public accounting firm Canada	Transportation company Ontario, Canada	Prince Edward Island (Canada) public service	Nipissing & Temiskaming Assessment referral service Ontario, Canada
Workforce Size	2,150	1,640	7,552	
EAP delivery	External	Internal	Internal	External/consortium
Study time-frame	one point in time	4 years	4 years	point-in-time interviews
Study's purpose	program use and satisfaction	employee & organization perspectives on EAP	program analysis for future planning	how does this model of EAP impact quality of life?
Methodology	anonymous organization-wide survey (n=1608)	• client survey (n = 101) • counsellor interviews • company records using a case-control design (for each EAP user a matched subject found)	• surveys: clients (n=81) employees (n=236) managers (n=53) manager's focus group (n=18) • 11 key informants • comparison with four other EAPs	Key-Informant Interviews • 9 worksites 5 individuals
Total methods used	1	3	4	1

(cont.)

Outcome			
• 78% aware of program • 60% would use program • 6% had used program and reported being somewhat satisfied with the program • 3.6–4.1 on 5 items with 4 indicating somewhat satisfied	• 89% of EAP users very satisfied • 66% indicated life has changed for the better • 2% worsened • job performance change: 21% improved a lot 25% improved slightly 44% stayed the same • EAP users have more sick days and compensation claims than non-users	• 61% of clients reported workplace problems pre-EAP use; 7% post • 54% replied EAP was a workplace necessity • overall satisfaction but more training, technical support and awareness programming needed • program needs to become more proactive	• ARS model intervenes with individual, family, work, and the community • ARS not only intervention but also a vehicle for community development • ARS builds cooperation between labour and management • focus on prevention & education, not only treatment • antithesis of managed care approach

Adapted from: Bennett, 1978; Burke, 1994; Chandler, Kroeker, Flynn & MacDonald, 1988; Groeneveld, Shain, Brayshaw & Heideman, 1984; Johnson, Docherty, Michalenko, Bucklee & Hazlett, 1989; Lindop, 1975; Lynch, 1980; Macdonald, Lothian & Wells, 1997; Mowry, Hogan, Moase, Montgomery & Harper, 1987; Ontario Addiction Research Foundation, 1990; Newman, 1983; Pergantes, 1982; Sargeant & Tepperman, 1987; Shain & Suurvali, 1997; Van Halm, 1998.

Csiernik, R. (1997). The relationship between program developers and delivery of occupational assistance. *Employee Assistance Quarterly* 13(2), 31–53.

Csiernik, R. (1998). A profile of Canadian Employee Assistance Programs. *Employee Assistance Research Supplement* 2(1), 1–8.

Groeneveld, J., Shain, M., Brayshaw, D., & Heideman, I. (1984). *The Alcoholism Treatment Program at Canadian National Railways.* Toronto: Addiction Research Foundation.

Jerrell, J. & Rightmyer, J. (1982). Evaluating Employee Assistance Programs: A review of methods, outcomes, and future directions. *Evaluation and Program Planning* 5(3), 255–267.

Johnson, P., Docherty, O., Michalenko, C., Bucklee, J., & Hazlett, J. (1989). REACHing out at Red Deer College. *EAP Digest* 9(3), 12, 53–54.

Kurtz, N., Googins, B., & Howard, W. (1984). Measuring the success of occupational alcoholism programs. *Journal of Studies on Alcohol* 45(1), 33–45.

Lindop, S. (1975). Three Canadian industrial alcoholism programs. In R. Williams and G. Moffat (eds.), *Occupational alcoholism programs.* Springfield: Charles C. Thomas.

Lynch, J. (1980). Variations in program usage in different occupational settings. *Labour–Management Alcoholism Journal* 10(3), 85–96.

Macdonald, S. (1986). *Evaluating EAPs.* Toronto: Addiction Research Foundation.

Macdonald, S., Lothian, S., & Wells, S. (1997). Evaluation of an Employee Assistance Program at a transportation company. *Evaluation and Program Planning* 20(4), 495–505.

Merriam, S. (1989). *Case study research in education.* San Francisco: Jossey-Bass.

Mowry, S., Hogan, S., Moase, O., Montgomery, D., & Harper, B. (1997). *Public sector Employee Assistance Program: Program evaluation.* Charlottetown: Government of Prince Edward Island.

Ontario Addiction Research Foundation. (1990). *Statistics on EAP utilization.* Toronto: Addiction Research Foundation.

Newman, P. (1983). Program evaluation as a reflection of program goals. In R. Thomlinson (ed.), *Perspectives on industrial social work practice.* Toronto: Family Service Canada.

Pergantes, B. (1982). *LEAC—A communal employee benefit business.* London: LEAC.

Rodriguez, J. & Borgen, W. (1998). Needs assessment: Western Canada's program administrators' perspectives on the role of EAPs in the workplace. *Employee Assistance Quarterly* 14(2), 11–29.

Sargeant, L. & Tepperman, P. (1987). People and profits at Central Canada Grocers: HR ventures into EAP monitoring software. *Human Resources Management in Canada.* Toronto: Prentice-Hall.

Shain, M. & Suurvali, H. (1997). *Feeding four birds with one hand: Results of the Nipissing/Temiskaming EFAP/ARS Impact Study.* Toronto: Addiction Research Foundation.

Tesch, R. (1990). *Qualitative research.* New York: Falmer Press.

US Department of Health and Human Services. (1986). *Standards and criteria for the development and evaluation of a comprehensive Employee Assistance Program.* Rockville, Maryland.

Van Halm, R. (1988). Out of the woods. *Occupational Health and Safety Canada* 4(6), 22–29.

Yin, R. (1989). *Case study research: Design and methods.* London: Sage.

Part III

PRACTICE

9

Assessment in
an EAP Environment

Frank MacAulay

Introduction

> Guess what? When it comes right down to it, wherever you go there you
> are. Whatever you wind up doing, that's what you've wound up doing.
> Whatever you are thinking right now, that's what's on your mind. Whatever
> has happened to you, it has already happened. The important question is
> how are you going to handle it? In other words, "Now what?"
>
> Jon Kabat-Zinn, 1994

In setting the stage for an Employee-Assistance professional to help an
employee address the question "Now what?," one must consider that the
environment of the Employee Assistance Program (EAP). The Employee-
Assistance counsellor must be familiar with the workplace context in
order to understand the dynamics that may be at play for the employee
as he[1] enters the EAP office. Having an active EAP Advisory Committee,
composed of representatives of labour and management, will help the
program counsellors understand the nature of the work environment from
both perspectives. This is easier to attain with internal programs, though
organizations that use external program providers can obtain similar
insights through the use of trained peer-referral agents, who can be of great
assistance to off-site program managers and counsellors. It is beneficial for
Employee-Assistance professionals to have regular contact with work-site
managers and human resource departments, in order to understand any
work-based cultural changes and the potential impact that these have on
employees. As Employee Assistance Programs mature, there is typically
an increasing number of supervisors who seek advice, consultation, and

assistance in dealing with stressful situations in the workplace. For example, the Province of Prince Edward Island's (2003) internal program has had as much as 20 percent of referrals arise as a result of supervisor suggestions or informal supervisory referrals.

The Supervisory Consultation and Assessment

Let us examine the supervisory consultation before we look at the employee entering the counsellor's office. The supervisor needs to view the EAP as a support and resource for managers; otherwise, she may not think of the service as an option when dealing with a difficult personnel situation. As well, the EAP Advisory Committee needs to market this feature as a key component of the program. When the supervisor calls, the EAP counsellor must allow as much time and privacy for the consultation as they would for an individual counselling session. A face-to-face consultation, rather than a phone conversation, helps the supervisor assess the impact of a given problem not only on the work unit, but also on the supervisor herself. In many situations, the supervisor is calling after "an event," and may be experiencing a range of emotions; this is an excellent entry for an EAP to discuss the impact of stress in the workplace. EAP counsellors need to discuss the range of supports available to the supervisor, ranging from general to specific training needs, including topics such as conducting supervisor-assisted referral and coping with stress or trauma. EAP service providers must also be sensitive to non-work issues that supervisors may be encountering, which may affect the objectivity of the circumstances at work. In certain situations, this supervisory consultation may easily and appropriately turn into a counselling session for the supervisor.

The EAP counsellor needs to explore options that the supervisor has tried, or is planning to try, in resolving the work-related issue. Avenues to explore include: has there been consultation with the union? Has there been discipline in the past, or is discipline a pending option? If there is job conflict, is mediation an option?[2] Part of this initial supervisory assessment process is to explore how, according to the supervisor, this problem may affect the employee's work, the supervisor, and the work unit. Often, the consultation also needs to explore whether an informal offer of assistance should be made to the employee, or whether the situation warrants a formal offer of assistance. Clarification of the role of EAP versus a substance-abuse assessment, a fit-for-duty assessment, or duty-to-accommodate assessment must also take place. These latter assessments are medically driven, generally governed by the collective agreement, and may not be voluntary; for this reason they are not part of the EAP service, and should not be directly associated with the services offered by EAP. However, the Employee Assistance Program may still typically have a role in these situations. It may be through collaborating with the employee and the employer in relation to these areas, or serving as a facilitator to finding an acceptable solution for all—but only with informed consent, and within the bounds of the principles of confidentiality (Canadian Employee Assistance Program Association, 1997).

As the supervisory consultation ends, it is hoped that the supervisor has developed a sense of the options available and optimal route to follow in addressing work-site stress, as well as realizing that EAP is there for ongoing support for both the supervisor and the employee, as well as for other members of the work unit, as required. It is also hoped that through this assessment process the EAP will develop a picture of the work unit, as well as identifying any EAP training and marketing needs for that work-site. Through these types of consultations, EAP usage will increase, as word-of-mouth is one of the primary ways EAP is propagated within a workplace.

First Contact

It is now time to consider the employee who is under an inordinate amount of stress, in crisis or uncertain where to turn in dealing with an overwhelming problem. What is his typical first contact with the organization's formal helping service? The initial contact by an employee who has never used EAP—or may not even be aware of exactly what EAP or counselling is—is a crucial step for introducing the service. Whoever receives that initial phone call or e-mail must reinforce the principles of the EAP: that contact, be it by phone or by e-mail, will be confidential, and that contact will never be made through an impersonal switchboard, call-display service, or general inquiry e-mail mailbox. In this way it is immediately demonstrated to the employee that they are using a secure and safe service.

The assigned counsellor, upon first contact, reviews the general nature of the situation in terms of mandate to, and the context of, the work-site, the nature of the joint union–management agreement, and the type of services offered by the EAP, including short-term counselling, critical incident stress debriefing, or family counselling. An enquiry is made about any concerns or questions the employee may have about the program. How the employee learned of the service is particularly useful both in terms of understanding how best to promote the program in the future, and also in supporting the referral route through which the employee accessed the EAP. There should always be a brief discussion of the principles of the program, again highlighting the core program components of confidentiality, neutrality, and the voluntary nature of the service. However, employees also need to be aware of the limits of confidentiality to which the EAP counsellor is bound by the laws of the province. They should also be aware of the specific circumstance under which certain information will have to be released: if, for example, it pertains to child abuse or harm to oneself or others. If the employee has accessed the EAP through a formal supervisory offer process, a discussion must take place to help the employee clearly understand the EAP relationship with the supervisor, and to reinforce the fact that no identifying information will be shared with the workplace. As well, the employee needs to clearly understand that the service is voluntary in nature, and that a formal process still entails voluntary participation on the employee's part (Canadian Employee Assistance Program Association, 1997). With this introduction to the service, the employee is ready to move into the "Now what?" stage of the assessment.

Assessing the Employee

When asking the employee to present an overview of why he is here now, many EAP counsellors hear, "I don't know where to begin." Many employees state that they have been thinking about their situation for some time, and could have been here months or even years ago. In this early beginning the EAP counsellor will obtain the sense of how the employee has been trying to manage using his own resources, before calling for help. The counsellor enquires whether the employee has ever contacted a counsellor before, and if so, the nature of the request and satisfaction with service. It is also important to clarify what satisfaction means to the employee, as it can potentially bias this relationship with the EAP counsellor. As well, male employees are generally not as comfortable identifying and sharing feelings as are females, particularly in male-dominated work sectors where EAPs are still more common; so the EAP counsellor needs to normalize the idea of talking about feelings.

To help the employee present a full picture of her situation, it is vital to "step gently" by having her first talk about work. By having her present a picture of her work world, the EAP counsellor can obtain an understanding of why this type of work was chosen, the length of time in this job or position, and how the employee adjusts to change—for all work-sites are dealing with change—and how the change has impacted the employee. During this discussion, value conflicts that may be present as a result of the changing work environment, and the way the employee is be coping with the difficulty may be uncovered; an assessment can be made of whether there are any connections to loss in other areas of the employee's life. By gaining an understanding of work habits—including punctuality, use of breaks, overtime, what the employee worries about at work, and what causes distraction at work—the EAP counsellor may obtain a picture of the employee's thoughts and feelings about herself in relation to her work world. In having the employee discuss relationships with co-workers, supervisors, and customers, the EAP counsellor develops a sense of the emotional connection to the work world. This will also provide a picture of the employee's ability to handle a variety of relationships, to deal with conflict, and to be committed to dealing with issues; it will also be a tool for identifying work relationships that trigger memories of unresolved personal relationships or past abusive relationships. It is important to have the employee reflect on the impact of her stress on her work, subjectively including such things as days missed because of not being able to cope, accidents because of preoccupied thoughts, and decrease in quality and quantity of work. It is also necessary to obtain an understanding of whether a co-worker or a supervisor has ever mentioned any of these behaviours to her, and if so, if there was ever any discipline as a result.

As the employee finishes his picture of his work world, it is important to obtain a sense of whether any part of work sparks the employee's real "spirit of being." Many employees are able to identify some project or activity that has real meaning for them, and it is valuable for them to think about how they will ensure that this can continue. It is helpful to obtain an understanding of what supports an employee may feel are present in the work environment. These could come from people such as supervisors, the human resources department, or co-workers; or they could come from the workplace environment itself, for example, having or setting up appropriate work space; or activities such as taking breaks, going for a walk, or setting realistic limits on time commitments and projects. Some employees quickly recognize that there is much support in their work world. If the employee is stating that he perceives few supports in terms of people, environment, or personal power within the work world, this will typically impact other areas of his life and also his wellness.

As the initial assessment continues, the EAP counsellor needs to have the employee slowly begin to share her story of her non-work life. During this portion of the opening session, the counsellor wants the employee to share the joys and hurts of her personal relationships. This includes gaining an understanding of her significant relationships, whether she is single, married, or in a same-sex partnership. As she shares her story of her present nuclear relationships, we gain an understanding of what her problem-solving abilities are, where she senses real contentment, where situations are in order, and where there is strain. The employee may wish to share significant stories from her extended family that have an impact on her present life. As well, she may come to realize where there are value conflicts within her family and how these are impacting her, or even potentially being replayed in the workplace. The EAP counsellor can also assist the employee to explore her social network: how money is managed, what she has for social activities/supports, exercise, hobbies, and interests. During this stage of the assessment the EAP counsellor obtains a sense of what keeps the employee going through her many issues. Through this conversation the employee is helped to identify the people, places, and things that are "energy fillers" and "energy drainers" in her personal life.

During this assessment process with the employee, the EAP counsellor needs to be aware of other areas in need of further exploration. This includes the whole area of use of addictive substances or compulsive behaviours that are used to cope with life events. Counsellors should also explore the key area of past and present trauma, including physical and/or sexual abuse, as there may be work relationships that are reminders of past abuse. For some employees, coming to the Employee Assistance Program is the first opportunity to identify the impact of past events on their life. It is important to help the employee accept the pain of past events, and to incorporate some reflections on how the employee may want to deal with the pain of addiction and/or abuse.

On many occasions, the EAP assessment interview is similar to a medical triage. The EAP practitioner will have to look at the stress-to-burn-out continuum with the employee: many arrive in a high state of anxiety and exhaustion or in an active crisis state. This continuum includes:

- helping the employee understand the range of her thought processes from experiencing worry and occasional fear to being cynical and pessimistic all the time;
- helping the employee understand her range of emotions, from being anxious, annoyed, and easily agitated; to being completely apathetic, lethargic, and unable to react emotionally; and,
- helping the employee look at behaviours, ranging from avoiding others, being indecisive, explosive, or belligerent; to a change in eating/sleeping patterns, withdrawing from work and personal contacts, and being resigned to failure.

Health issues that employees will report along this continuum range from concern about anxiety to heart attacks to various stages of depression. When an individual has become completely overwhelmed by all of life's issues, and has moved beyond burn-out, suicide ideation can oftentimes occur. The EAP counsellor needs to assess the risk for follow-through, and then develop a safety plan, including contracting with the client, if necessary.

This entire assessment process assists the employee to obtain a picture of his "energy balance": an understanding of the energy used in dealing with work and personal issues, and the amount of energy expended to minimize the impact on work, family, and self. Having the employee diagram a "pie of life" in terms of energy used in all activities in his/her life will help him/her visualize the balance or imbalance in his/her personal wellness, and where adjustments may need to be made.

The counsellor needs to be skilled in helping the employee differentiate between situational stress and physical/mental exhaustion and depression. At this time, some type of communication may need to take place between the employee and her supervisor. The employee needs to know that some employers have difficulty with the words "stress" and "stress leave"; and the EAP counsellor needs to help the employee determine the most appropriate information to provide the employer, without isolating the physician, who remains critical to this process; and without breaching confidentiality with any health-care provider.

Some employees come to realize that they are so physically and mentally exhausted that they must take medical leave from work in order to start rebuilding their lives. They have come to believe that they have no personal power over anything at this stage, and therefore need to take time off to rebuild confidence in themselves in their personal lives, before addressing the work issues that brought them to the EAP. Generally there is much anxiety about taking "stress" leave, so it is important to help employees explore how they are currently functioning and what choices they have, considering their physical and emotional functioning. It is extremely important to ensure the employee is able to make a comfortable decision about personal or medical stress leave: at times of stress, our ability to make decisions is even further constricted, and we may want others to decide for us.

As the assessment winds down, the EAP counsellor needs to help the employee identify the "Gas Stations of Life"—those supports, ever so small, that will help the employee move ahead and regain control of his life. Upon reflection, the employee will come to realize that many of these supports come from the "I used to walk, swim, sing, play cards ..."—small activities that provided contentment, joy, and a sense of what was important for him. He will come to realize that he can access some of these supports that were helpful in the past.

Concluding the Assessment

It is important to obtain the employee's perceptions of his/her major issues through the course of the assessment process. The EAP counsellor needs to summarize the perceived impact of these issues on an individual employee's thought process in terms of his or her intellectual health, on the employee's emotions and spiritual health, and on the employee's behaviours. There are physical and social components to wellness. Through this the employee will have a better understanding of stress, its impact on her life balance, and the amount of energy used to maintain a balance point. The summary at the conclusion of the assessment includes identifying the employee's hopes and goals, areas where she can start to exercise some control and personal power, and helping her to plan around the available options. The EAP counsellor needs to discuss with the employee what options for assistance are available under the auspices of the program, and what may need to be referred to outside community resources. A discussion of post-service evaluation, including providing an evaluation form for feedback, needs to take place in this initial assessment. Release-of-information forms may also need to be completed to allow contact with collateral individuals or organizations such as the supervisor, community agencies, doctors, and related social and health services. Many employees also look for homework assignments, which can begin the process of personal power development; therefore a discussion should also follow about independent work and tasks, when an employee begins to take small steps towards personal recovery. Finally, when possible, the EAP should develop a resource library as many individuals will request articles, handouts, or books to read, to further enhance their understanding of their situation. There are also a number of stress-management tools such as the StressMap, Myers Briggs Type Inventory, and Insights Discovery, that will provide the employee with a visual and concrete understanding of herself. These too can become valuable components of the employee's personal recovery plan.

Lastly, it is important to ask the employee how this session was helpful in addressing the "Now what?" that brought him to EAP. The EAP assessment will have covered a number of areas in helping the employee set his course. There will be an increased awareness of what the stressors are in his life, and the impact they are having on him physically, emotionally, and cognitively; a beginning acceptance of what this has done to him and those who are close to him; relief in being able to share what is happening, a feeling of relief that has both physical and emotional components. There will also be a beginning hope that he will be able to start moving through his pain; and a commitment to answering the "Now what?" himself each moment he encounters it along his journey.

Endnotes

1. Female and male pronouns will be used interchangeably in this chapter.
2. See Chapter 17 for a further discussion of mediation services.

References

Canadian Employee Assistance Program Association. (1997). *Practice standards and guidelines.* Saskatoon: CEAPA.

Kabat-Zinn, J. (1994). *Wherever you go there you are.* Toronto: Hyperion.

Province of Prince Edward Island. (2003). *Annual statistical report.* Charlottetown.

10

Crisis Intervention
in the EAP Context

Susan Alexander

Introduction

Many are surprised to learn that Dukkha, the first Noble Truth in Buddhist teaching, is interpreted by most scholars to represent the Buddhist belief that all of life is suffering. This is far from a pessimistic view; rather, Buddhism suggests we accept that life is difficult and that it is filled with pain and obstacles. Buddhist philosophy would encourage us to adopt a realistic, rather than overly optimistic, view of the journey of life, and release ourselves from attachment to expectations of a life free from challenges and crisis. In accepting this truth, we are better able to prepare for and rise above the suffering which will be experienced throughout life (Rahula, 1959).

Intermittent suffering that often leads to an acute crisis state can be thought of as part of the normal human condition. Few people will be fortunate enough to avoid crisis moments in their lifetime. Based on this view, it is appropriate to suggest that many of the clients we will see within the Employee Assistance Program (EAP) context will encounter challenging life experiences and will seek relief and guidance in resolving barriers to their life's goals. This is, often, where we meet our clients' most intense and immediate need: when they are experiencing a state of crisis.

Although most people, when asked, would view crisis in their lives as a negative occurrence, many crisis theorists have described this situation as an opportunity. The symbol in the Chinese language for crisis represents both danger and opportunity (Gilliland & James, 2001; Kanel, 2003). Danger is present in the sense that most people in crisis often have an overwhelming fear of loss of a significant part of their life, past, present, or future. The client experiences a wide range of reactions which may include extreme thoughts such as self-harm or harm to others. Opportunity is represented in the change that crisis can present in one's life, and the coping that may lead to the development of adaptive skills in managing future crises. Inherent in this description of crisis is the belief that crisis can represent a breakthrough for an individual. It can be a turning point and an opportunity for change.

Crisis Theory: A Brief History

Many prominent clinical theorists contributed to the foundations of crisis theory and intervention, including Freud and Erikson (Aguilera, 1998; Bellak & Small, 1965; Erikson, 1963; Rappaport, 1959); however it is the research and clinical interventions of Eric Lindemann that are considered to have the most significant impact in contemporary crisis work (Lindemann, 1995; Roberts, 1991). Lindemann and his associates from Massachusetts General Hospital studied the reactions of the survivors and surviving family members of the Coconut Grove Nightclub fire, an event which occurred in Boston, Massachusetts in November, 1942. The fire was a tragic incident believed to be caused by a lit match that ignited highly flammable decorations in the nightclub. It is estimated that the capacity of the club was nearly triple its acceptable limit on this night, and approximately 493 people perished in the confusion and panic. Lindemann's study in the aftermath of this horrific event focused on psychological and acute grief reactions of those closely related to the deceased fire victims. The findings in this research provided crisis theory with a foundation of understanding that grief work requires certain stages of mourning and eventual acceptance of the experienced loss. Without progression through these stages, an individual is likely to encounter a crisis reaction in a more acute state at some point in the future (Lindemann, 1995). Gerald Caplan (1964) further expanded on Lindemann's work and was the first psychiatrist to study the concept of homeostatis as it relates to the stages of crisis (Roberts, 1991). Caplan also identified the opportunity inherent in a crisis to develop improved or worsened emotional coping. Depending on the adaptive or maladaptive response to the crisis, the individual would likely carry forward this response to future crisis experiences. Caplan thus provided us with the understanding that effective crisis intervention is not only restorative but also preventative (Caplan, 1964; Turner, 1996).

Types of Crises

Our clients seek support from the EAP when they feel they do not have the capacity to resolve the problems in their lives by utilizing their usual coping mechanisms and resources. Many types of situations may cause an employee or family member to contact the EAP; the most frequent often involve either a situational or developmental crisis. Developmental crises occur when, in the process of normal transitions between developmental stages, as identified by Erikson, the individual experiences an inability to cope with the transition and the demands or expectations of the next developmental stage (Kanel, 2003). For example, a developmental crisis may occur when a new mother is having difficulty coping with the demands of a newborn child, or when a long-term employee begins thinking of retirement. In contrast, a situational crisis, according to Caplan (1964), is primarily environmental and often involves loss of some kind, such as the loss of basic needs for love, or loss of bodily integrity. A situational crisis is typically an uncommon event that an individual has no way of anticipating (Caplan, 1964; Gilliland & James, 2001). These events might include a sexual assault, the sudden death of a child, or a plant closing unexpectedly. Defining client crisis in one category or another may assist the counsellor in determining an intervention plan, though it is also of value to assess if a client is experiencing several different crises concurrently.

Crisis Intervention versus Brief Therapy

Short-term, solution-focused, brief work tends to be the basis for much of EAP activity. Brief therapy and task-centred therapy have many similar therapeutic approaches to crisis intervention, such as:

- maintaining clear goals
- enhanced counsellor activity
- time limits
- a focus on client and other resources outside of the therapeutic relationship
- ongoing evaluation and flexibility of treatment
- alternative concepts of session time and place, and
- specifically planned follow-up (Cournoyer, 1996).

Though many clients present in crisis and EAP counsellors may engage with them within a brief-therapy model, crisis work differs in intent from this practice.

Crisis intervention is time-limited, usually no more that six weeks in duration, and sessions must be scheduled to ensure that the EAP counsellor has adequate time to ensure client safety. This may entail, for example, staying with a client who may be suicidal or homicidal until adequate support can be arranged. Crisis work is also single-issue focused, targeting the precipitating crisis and related subjective distress of the client, and relies on setting realistic goals that are limited in scope. If additional issues are identified, the counsellor and employee need to work together to develop alternative plans for those issues. Expectations of major transformations will lead to frustration for both the counsellor and employee or family member. Treatment focuses on assisting the client in returning to their pre-crisis level of functioning (Myer, 2001).

Crisis intervention specifically seeks to assist the client in identifying and ameliorating distortions in subjective perception brought on by a precipitating event. These distortions include affective, behavioural, and cognitive responses that are often temporary and quite resolvable (Gilliland & James, 2001). The overarching goal of crisis intervention is to assist the individual in regaining a sense of equilibrium and homeostasis to a pre-crisis level of functioning.

Process of a Crisis

It is generally accepted by the current literature that the stages of escalating crisis are as follows:

i)   A stressful precipitating event occurs, which is meaningful or threatening to the individual; the individual experiences subjective distress, and psychological disorganization/disequilibrium ensues;
ii) An attempt is made by the individual to manage the event, and this may be either adaptive or maladaptive, in terms of previously experienced or observed coping methods. These methods are either satisfactory in resolving the crisis (the crisis state diminishes), or these methods fail to produce the desired results in changing or resolving the crisis;
iii) The subjective distress increases when the employee realizes that known, previously successful coping methods are inadequate to resolve this crisis. Thus, the person is left functioning at a lower psychological, behavioural, and emotional level than at the pre-crisis state and feels even more threatened, with disequilibrium increasing. (Kanel, 2003; Parad & Parad, 1990; Roberts, 1990).

Crisis Occurs in the Eye of the Beholder

In order to develop a plan of intervention, the most important aspect of understanding an employee in crisis is, as much as possible, seeing the crisis as he or she views it. Although we seek to understand our client's experience in the majority of therapeutic models, crisis intervention is unique. The subjective nature of the client's reaction at a time when their cognitive processes are in disarray requires additional skills on the part of EAP counsellors to narrow their focus on the meaning of the crisis to the individual client. Employees' usual thought processes are often disorganized, and the psychological impact of the precipitating event can be difficult for them to comprehend and for the counsellor to assess. Typically, an EAP counsellor will need to manage or change the client's internal experience of the precipitating event, rather than co-opting with the client in crisis, who may be more focused on the details of the event itself (Kanel, 2003).

Assessment is critical in identifying the subjective experience of the crisis for the client; however, the nature of crisis intervention precludes many advantages available in brief- or long-term therapy. Clearly defining the scope of the problem, discussing alternative solutions with the client, and developing methodological plans are more constrained in crisis intervention by the fact that clients need to stabilize quickly, often in one or two sessions (Gilliland & James, 2001). Assessment is crucial in effective crisis intervention and often must be done quickly (Myer, 2001). Inaccurate assessment can lead to destructive psychological disturbances in the individual's coping with the crisis, and can be disastrous if the client is thinking of harming him or herself or others.

Comprehensive crisis assessment includes identifying the client's affect, behaviour, and cognitive functioning (Myer, 2001) in order to plan intervention effectively. Abnormal affect can also be assessed by being sensitive to the client's emotional stance and by determining if the client's emotional presentation is congruent with the precipitating event. Behavioural response can be assessed by observing the client's psychomotor activity, and in his or her role in taking active steps in responding to the crisis. Immobility can represent a feeling of disempowerment and a sense of diminished control. It is both helpful and important to assist the client in remembering previously successful crisis and coping mechanisms to encourage forward thinking. Cognitive functioning, although more difficult to assess quickly, is primary to understanding the meaning that the client attaches to the precipitating event. Observing the level of client's realism and consistency in relation to the crisis is helpful, as is determining whether the client is rationalizing or minimizing the event, or appropriately assessing the impact of this event in their life (Gilliland & James, 2001).

Professional Stance in Crisis Intervention

It is important to consider the effect that the EAP counsellor will have in managing the crisis experience with the client. When engaging a client who interprets their situation as overwhelming, hopeless, disempowering, and impossible to control, the counsellor represents a stabilizing force in this experience. Thus, professional presence and stance are important in conveying many verbal and non-verbal messages to the client. Important characteristics of effective crisis workers include life experience, professional skills, poise, creativity, and flexibility. A calm presence is imperative, particularly in situations where the client is violent or physically compromised by the crisis experience. One can achieve such a presence by attending to client's needs for physical space, using a calm and soothing voice to address the client, using gestures and body language to slow the client's agitated state, and demonstrating through one's demeanour a comfort level with client's need to express his or her feelings to the fullest range, while maintaining a safe therapeutic environment (Gilliland & James, 2001).

Working through a crisis situation with a client requires a great deal of focus on the client as well as attention to our own reactions and needs. Crisis intervention is intense work; it can be exhausting and stressful. Crisis intervention demands that the counsellor's collective experience and skill be on full alert and ready at a moment's notice for use. Like in other therapeutic models, experience in crisis intervention allows for a comfort level to develop with the intensity, pace, and advanced skills that are demanded. It is helpful to remember that your specific goal is to assist the client in stabilizing to their pre-crisis level of functioning, and all efforts in crisis intervention need be directed to that goal.

The therapeutic challenges can be better managed with good supports in place for those who engage with clients in crisis. Trusted supervision, peer consultation, opportunities for non-crisis-oriented work, and a good knowledge of the counsellor's personal reaction to crisis situations are essential in maintaining balance within crisis work.

Crisis Intervention Models

Developing and maintaining rapport with a client in crisis are essential in communicating understanding and trustworthiness. When a client feels unable to rely upon pass, and otherwise trusted, coping methods, it is imperative that the counsellor create a climate in which the client can feel safe and free to disclose his or her fears about the crisis. The nature of crisis intervention is such that the development of rapport often needs to occur quickly and without detail of information; and also often without the opportunity for the client to develop a comfort level with the EAP counsellor. Basic attending skills of eye contact, warm presence, body posture, vocal style, verbal following, and client-focused empathy will help the client tell their story in an environment where they can trust they will be heard and helped (Kanel, 2003).

Several prominent crisis-intervention models are available to the EAP practitioner for use. However, determining your own process in engaging a client in crisis will develop much like your own therapeutic model(s) and essence. Crisis-intervention models provide us with a structure and process to guide us when supporting people who are feeling intense emotional response, which includes feeling numb, and where situations in counselling can become out of control. When first engaging in crisis intervention work, you may find it helpful to use the models available to reflect back on your practice in order to identify opportunities for improvement.

Kanel (2003) developed a comprehensive three-part ABC Model of Crisis Intervention which combines many components of current crisis-intervention practice and which is also readily applicable to an EAP environment. The ABC model's three components are:

A: developing and maintaining rapport
B: identifying the problem
C: coping

A: Developing and maintaining rapport

As mentioned earlier, developing and maintaining rapport are essential in providing the EAP client with an atmosphere of emotional safety and understanding. The ABC model postulates which this can be facilitated through the use of communication skills that support rapport-building, including the use of attending behaviour, appropriate use of open-ended and closed-ended questions, paraphrasing, reflection of feelings, and summarization (Ivey, 1999; Kanel, 2003). Use of these communication skills allows EAP practitioners to assist clients in feeling understood while simultaneously calming the situation by helping clients in organize their information. It also allows the client to feel empowered by answering fact-based questions, while encouraging the employee or family member to express feelings about the presenting crisis situation (Kanel, 2003).

B: Identifying the poblem

Many clients, both employees and family members, who present in crisis to EAP counsellors need little prompting to describe the precipitating event for which they are seeking. Assisting the client in organizing the information provided enables the counsellor to more accurately identify the underlying issue in the crisis: the client's subjective distress. The client will undoubtedly identify the problem as the precipitating event itself, and perhaps find that it is a significant obstacle. Maintaining the focus of the sessions with the client on their cognitive interpretation provides the EAP practitioner with a direction to reduce clients' subjective distress and implement new or enhanced coping skills, thus enabling clients to access a higher level of psychological functioning (Kanel, 2003). The ABC Model offers several suggestions to assist a counsellor in uncovering the cognitive interpretation of the event with the client. These are not presented as a linear process but rather as a list of suggestions for assessing this aspect of the crisis for the client by weaving together these key areas. The pieces are:

- identifying the precipitating event;
- exploring cognitions;
- identifying emotional distress;
- identifying impairments in behavioural, social, intellectual, and occupational functioning;
- identifying the pre-crisis level of functioning;
- identifying ethical issues such as suicide assessment, child abuse, elder abuse, danger to others, organic or other medical concerns;
- identifying substance abuse issues; and,
- using therapeutic interactions: educational, empowerment, supportive comments, and reframes (Kanel, 2003: 41).

Until the EAP practitioner is able to unlock the door to the client's understanding and cognitive interpretation of the precipitating event, the process cannot move forward to intervention. To do so would risk inappropriate and misguided intervention, which could fail to address the need of the client, and which puts the client at risk of concretizing poor responses to future crises.

C: Coping

When working with a client in crisis, the counsellor may experience the temptation to address only current attempts at coping with the situation. It is, however, imperative that the client be provided the opportunity to take a step back from the current crisis to examine successful coping in the past, to consider attempts to manage this present crisis, and to consider coping attempts in the future. Any attempt on the part of the employee or family member to identify successful coping in the past, both within and outside of the workplace environment, should be commended and used as a foundation for building the crisis-intervention plan. The client also benefits from understanding that even some maladaptive coping mechanisms have short-term benefits. For example, temporary social withdrawal can be reframed as an attempt to manage the overwhelming impact of the external stimuli when the client is already feeling overwhelmed, and may have been helpful in stabilizing the client while they were debating seeking out professional support.

Assisting clients in identifying their coping behaviours and building awareness around the continuum of appropriate application is helpful in self-regulating their crisis response in the future; in other words, creating a kind of internal gauge. This also provides an opportunity for the EAP practitioners, particularly those who are internal to the organization, to encourage clients to develop new environment-related coping behaviours that they may have not considered. It is also important for the counsellor to be up-to-date on available community supports in order to assist clients in expanding their learning in this crisis. Services such as community groups aimed at psycho-educational process, support groups (or longer-term therapy that might address some additional issues identified in crisis intervention), agency-specific supports, medical, and legal referrals (Kanel, 2003) can provide the next appropriate step for clients to continue with this journey of understanding themselves in the presence of cognitively threatening life circumstances. An effective plan of intervention will seek commitment from the client to follow through on the coping suggestions, and will also include a formal, planned follow-up with the EAP counsellor at a mutually agreed-upon future point.

A Final Thought

Working with clients in crisis puts us in touch with raw and primitive emotions and reactions. It is real; the human condition in its most base state. In stepping forward and meeting clients at this point, we are provided the opportunity to connect with another's suffering. As such, we observe and experience suffering, too. As a counsellor or peer support, we must pay attention to the personal and professional toll that this process takes on us. It is helpful to adopt a spiritual component in crisis work; an understanding of the larger picture of crisis in human experience and an understanding of our limits within crisis work. Although the world is full of suffering, the world is also full of examples of human strength and survival, of overcoming and rediscovering hope.

This Work
Ken Kraybill, MSW

exhilarating and exhausting

drives me up a wall and opens doors I never imagined

lays bare a wide range of emotions yet leaves me feeling numb beyond
    belief

provides tremendous satisfaction and leaves me feeling profoundly
    helpless

evokes genuine empathy and provokes a fearsome intolerance within me
puts me in touch with deep suffering and points me toward greater
    wholeness
brings me face to face with many poverties and enriches me encounter
    by encounter
renews my hope and leaves me grasping for faith
enables me to envision a future but with no ability to control it
breaks me apart emotionally and breaks me open spiritually
leaves me wounded and
heals
me

References

Aguilera, D. (1998). *Crisis intervention: Theory and methodology.* St. Louis: Mosby
    Publishing.

Bellak, L. & Small, L. (1965). *Emergency psychotherapy and brief psychotherapy.* New
    York: Grune & Stratton.

Caplan, G. (1964). *Principles of preventive psychiatry.* New York: Basic Books.

Cournoyer, B. (1996). Crisis management and brief therapy. In A. Roberts (ed.),
    Crisis intervention handbook. Chicago: Nelson-Hall.

Eriskon, E. (1963). *Childhood and society* (2nd edn). New York: W.W. Norton.

Gilliland, B. & James, R. (2001). *Crisis intervention strategies* (4th edn). Belmont,
    California: Wadsworth.

Ivey, A. (1999). *Intentional interviewing and counselling: Facilitating client development in
    a multicultural world* (4th edn). Pacific Grove, California: Brooks Cole.

Kanel, K. (2003). *A guide to crisis intervention* (2nd edn). Belmont, California:
    Wadsworth.

Lindemann, E. (1995). *Crisis intervention.* Northvale, New Jersey: Aronson.

Myer, R. (2001). *Assessment for crisis intervention: A triage assessment model.* Belmont,
    California: Wadsworth.

Parad, H. & Parad, L. (1990). *Crisis intervention, Book 2: The practitioner's sourcebook
    for brief therapy.* Milwaukee, Wisconsin: Family Service America.

Rahula, W. (1959). *What the Buddha taught.* New York: Grove Weidenfeld.

Rappaport, D. (1959). A historical survey of psychoanalytic ego psychology.
    In G. Klein (ed.), *Psychological issues.* New York: International Universities
    Press.

Roberts, A. (1991). *Contemporary perspectives on crisis intervention and prevention.*
    Englewood Cliffs, New Jersey: Prentice-Hall.

Turner, F. (1996). *Social work treatment* (4th edn). New York: Free Press.

11

Critical Incident
Stress Management

Dermot Hurley, Sandy Ferreira, and Clare Pain

Introduction

Critical Incident Stress Management (CISM) is a comprehensive multimodal form of crisis management that evolved from earlier crisis-intervention models (Mitchell, 1983; Raphael, 1986). It was designed originally for emergency personnel who required a method of psychological debriefing to deal with the impact of exposure to critical incidents, which they witnessed in the course of their daily work. CISM has since expanded in scope and diversity of use, and is among the leading intervention models around the world for crisis-care workers and related personnel. According to Everly and Mitchell (1997), "CISM represents an integrated, comprehensive multicomponent crisis intervention program that spans the complete crisis continuum from the precrisis and acute crisis phases through the postcrisis phase." CISM is typically made available to individuals or groups immediately following a crisis, or in the aftermath of a crisis. The goals of CISM are twofold. The first is to restore individuals to their pre-crisis level of functioning, and the second is to arrest the development of maladaptive responses, which commonly occur as individuals attempt to come to terms with the critical incident, in particular Post Traumatic Stress Disorder [PTSD]. CISM has expanded to encompass organizations such as the military, airlines, banking, and recreational occupations. It is used in hospital settings to assist employees in the aftermath of a patient assault and in industry after an industrial accident or death.[1]

This chapter outlines the main components of CISM, focusing particularly on the process of psychological debriefing (CISD), and offers a brief review of the main studies related to outcomes. Critical Incident Stress Debriefing (CISD) is a term often used interchangeably with CISM, but refers in fact to one part of a multi-component intervention system which is more ambitious and wide reaching in scope. CISD is based on crisis theory and psycho-educational theory and is a key component in the seven core components of Critical Incident Stress Management described in Table 11.1 below. Much of the evaluative work on CISM has been conducted on the Mitchell CISD model and the majority of this chapter will focus on the CISD component of the CISM approach (Everly, Flannery, & Mitchell, 2000).

A Background to Critical Incident Stress Debriefing

One of the most widely used forms of crisis debriefing is Critical Incident Stress Debriefing, proposed by Mitchell in1983. In general the debriefing is not intended to be an intervention that stands on its own; rather, it should be considered one component of a comprehensive, integrated crisis-response program (Mitchell & Everly, 1993). The debriefing component of CISM is a tool used to facilitate a therapeutic discussion of individual thoughts and feelings following exposure to or involvement in a serious or distressing event. The formal process of CISD follows a structured seven-phase group meeting or discussion, whereby those who have been affected by the traumatic event are allowed the opportunity "to talk about their thoughts and emotions in a controlled and rational manner" (Everly, Lating, & Mitchell, 2000). The process is "designed to mitigate the psychological impact of a traumatic event and accelerate recovery from acute symptoms of distress that may arise in the immediate wake of a crisis or traumatic event" (Everly, Lating, & Mitchell, 2000). As crises impact larger numbers of individuals in society, crisis debriefing is rapidly becoming "one of the most popular approaches for dealing with trauma in groups of individuals affected by the same event. Several variations or models of debriefings have been described in the literature. CISD is the oldest and most widely utilized model and is often referred to as the 'Mitchell model' of debriefing" (Everly, Boyle, & Lating, 1999). An alternative debriefing process is the Raphael model and is similar in many respects to Mitchell's CISD, though it varies in certain aspects of content and process (Raphael, 1986; Regeher, 2001).

Critical Incident

Mitchell (1983) initially defined a critical incident as "any situation faced by emergency service personnel that causes them to experience unusually strong emotional reactions and has the potential to interfere with their ability to function either at the scene or later." As the definition of critical incident has evolved, more recently it has been defined as "any action that causes extraordinary emotion and overwhelms an individual's normal ability

Table 11.1: Critical Incident Stress Management (CISM): The seven core components

Intervention	Timing	Activation	Goals	Format
1. Precrisis preparation	Precrisis phase	Anticipation of crisis	Set expectations; improve coping	Groups Organizations
2. Individual crisis intervention (1:1)	Any time	Symptom-driven	Symptom mitigation; return to function, if possible; referral, if needed; stress mgmt.	Individuals
Large groups: 3a. Demobilizations & staff consult. (rescuers); 3b. Group info. briefing for schools, businesses, and large civilian groups	Shift disengagement; or, any time postcrisis	Event-driven	To inform, and consult; to allow for psychological decompression; stress management	Large groups Organizations
4. Critical Incident Stress Debriefing (CISD)	Postcrisis (1-10 days; at 3-4 weeks for mass disasters)	Usually symptom-driven; can be event-driven	Facilitate psychological closure; symptom mitigation; triage	Small groups
5. Defusing	Postcrisis (within 12 hrs)	Usually symptom-driven	Symptom mitigation; possible closure; triage	Small groups
Systems: 6a. Family CISM; 6b. Organizational consultation	Any time	Either symptom-driven or event-driven	Foster support, communications; symptom mitigation; closure, if possible; referral, if needed	Families Organizations
7. Follow-up; referral	Any time	Usually symptom-driven	Assess mental status; access higher level of care	Individual Family

Source: Everly & Mitchell (1999).

to cope, either immediately following the incident or in the future" (Conroy, 1990). It has been expanded further to include the idea of "a stressor event that has the potential to lead to a crisis response in many individuals" (Everly, 1999). The emphasis of the definition is both on the uniqueness of the events and the particular response of the individual, though it seems clear that critical incidents are typically "powerful and overwhelming incidents that lie outside the range of usual human experience" (Bell, 1995). The broadening of the definition of "critical incident" recognizes that such incidents are not simply isolated events, which target and impact specific at-risk populations, such as emergency personnel. Instead, these incidents can occur during the course of regular daily work or non-work activity, and have the potential to put a variety of people in different occupational situations at risk of experiencing traumatic reactions. Thus programs that include trauma-debriefing services can be applied to very diverse groups of people and employees.

When CISD first began, emergency personnel benefited from the opportunity to discuss the traumatic images and feelings evoked as they placed their own lives at risk. Without immediate access to professionals who conduct psychological debriefings, emergency personnel had difficulty facing the disturbing conditions to which they were exposed. It became obvious that many related occupational groups were affected by critical events, and researchers stressed the importance of debriefing in health-care environments in which the delivery of service to others might be jeopardized (Spitzer & Burke, 1993). In recent years, the use of CISD has expanded and, as already suggested, is no longer limited to healthcare and emergency personnel: it is now recognized that crises affect an increasingly large number of individuals in society.

Since critical incidents are not isolated events, no matter where they occur they not only impact those directly involved but also have the potential to impact hundreds of others (Miller, 2001). Incidents at schools, such as the Columbine shooting, affect not only the students, teachers, and staff present, but the local community as well as school personnel across the country (Miller, 2001). Moreover, the media's capacity to instantly transmit live first-hand accounts of disasters also contributes to spreading the impact of critical-incident events to an ever-expanding audience of potentially traumatized people. Terrorist attacks, such as the bombing of the World Trade buildings in New York (September 11, 2001), the subway bombings in Madrid (April 2004), and the school hostages and death of over 300 children and adults in Beslan, Russia (September 2004) have all created the conditions in which very large numbers of individuals are directly impacted by traumatic events.

Furthermore, children and adolescents have increasingly been identified as being at risk for experiencing traumatic events and their effects. For instance, adolescents who have experienced life-threatening situations such as car wrecks, disasters (both natural and man-made), or have been victims of rape, assault, or robbery can also benefit from CISD (Kirk & Madden, 2003). Although a full-scale debriefing may not be appropriate for use with children, it is important to note that the model can be adapted for children under 12 (Everly and Mitchell, 2000).

Symptoms

Regardless of how frequently traumatic events occur and how accustomed we become to witnessing them, the effects of exposure can still have a profound impact on individuals and groups. Symptoms of stress associated with critical incidents can often encompass serious physiological, behavioural, cognitive, and emotional reactions (Everly, 1990; Mitchell & Bray, 1990; Spitzer & Burke, 1993). Sleep disturbances, dizziness, migraines, and increased blood pressure are some of the physical concerns associated with exposure to a critical incident, while withdrawal, hyper-vigilance or excessive changes in activity, communication, or interaction may be some of the behavioural changes experienced following a critical event (Spitzer & Neely,1992). Stress triggered by the incident often results in cognitive impairment—poor concentration, confusion, difficulties in solving problems and making decisions, flashbacks—while emotionally the individual may experience profound depression, fear, increased levels of anxiety, guilt, or anger (van der Kolk, 1987; Gist & Lubin, 1989; Mitchell & Bray, 1990). Longer-term responses, particularly PTSD, have been associated with people who have been exposed to critical incidents; at this point, however, the extent to which stress and psychosocial factors are involved is unclear.

A tool such as CISD, within the CISM framework, which allows individuals the opportunity to discuss their thoughts and emotions in response to unusual circumstances, in theory should be highly beneficial in aiding those struggling to resolve individual reactions to an event. As well, the information gained during a debriefing about individual responses and various means of coping might provide some immediate relief and an understanding of normal reactions. The debriefing intervention may also encourage more adaptive responses in individuals, and also reduce the likelihood of developing more serious or complex stress reactions.

Post-traumatic stress is typically a normal response to an extreme event, usually followed by a normal recovery process. Chronic PTSD develops when the normal recovery process fails in some way, when the individual is unable to assimilate the experience and the acute symptoms intensify or persist (Campfield & Hills, 2001). Many factors have been identified as significant in the development of PTSD following exposure to trauma, which may have an impact on the overall effectiveness of CISD. Research has pointed to a number of key variables, including previous exposure, the severity and duration of the event, post-trauma experiences, and individual perceptions during and after the traumatic event (McFarlane & Yehuda, 1996). The debate about whether CISD is helpful in preventing the development of PTSD continues: recent studies argue that there has been insufficient research on psychological debriefing to substantiate this claim (Rose & Bisson, 1998). The mediating role of CISD in the prevention or onset of later PTSD remains unclear, and this subject will be explored later in the section on research findings (p. 163).

Response Time and Crisis Theory

The emphasis on time in critical-incident debriefing relates to a fundamental premise of crisis intervention[2] that requires that the intervention be applied within a specific time frame. Rapoport's (1967) conceptualization of crisis-intervention practice focused on the initial assessment period. She argued that to help someone in crisis, the individual must have rapid access to the worker: "a little help, rationally directed ... at a strategic time, is more effective than more extensive help given at a period of less emotional accessibility." The principles of crisis theory provide a rationale for the immediacy of debriefing sessions following a traumatic experience. The quick delivery of CISD following critical or traumatic incidents makes it a highly goal-oriented intervention. One of its main objectives is "to accelerate the recovery of individuals suffering from normal but painful realities to abnormal events" (Spitzer & Burke, 1993). The structured sessions that may last up to three hours are conducted 24 to 72 hours following a critical incident and involve confidential discussions of stress-provoking material. Conducting the debriefing to the affected persons within 72 hours of the event helps minimize the possibility that they will misinterpret their own personal reactions and become vulnerable to post-traumatic stress disorder (Spitzer & Burke, 1993). One study on the efficacy of CISD pointed to the beneficial results obtained by the immediate use of CISD following a crisis incident and fewer symptoms were reported in group members as a result (Campfield & Hills, 2001).

Mitchell's Model

The CISD component of Mitchell's comprehensive CISM model is composed of seven phases: an Introductory Phase, Fact-Finding Phase, Thought Phase, Reaction Phase, Symptom Phase, Teaching Phase, and

Re-entry Phase (Everly, Lating, & Mitchell, 2000). In the Introductory phase, facilitators begin by introducing themselves and briefly explaining to participants the purpose of the group. During this phase the tone for the debriefing is established, and it is important for the facilitators to be clear about the intent and process of the debriefing. Attendees are reassured that the symptoms they are experiencing are for the most part normal reactions to abnormal events (Mitchell & Bray, 1990). Only individuals directly affected are permitted to attend and are encouraged to speak, although there is no formal expectation to do so. Confidentiality is insured from the beginning, and guidelines, such as speaking only for oneself, are addressed in this phase. As well, no breaks are taken during the debriefing, and if a group member must leave the session, a debriefing team member accompanies them, to ensure that the member is not in any distress. It is particularly important in work-related situations that the employee be assured that participation in the debriefing will not result in disciplinary actions or impact his/her work evaluation. As well, it is important to reiterate that rank and position within an organization are irrelevant during a debriefing to further create a safe atmosphere for all participants to feel comfortable in engaging in the process (Spitzer & Neely, 1992).

In the Fact-Finding Phase each individual has a chance to explain the facts of the event from his or her own perspective. The exact order of events is irrelevant; instead each employee is given the opportunity to identify their role and responsibilities, and to explain how these duties contributed to their current reaction. By recounting what happened, the group members recreate the circumstances of the critical event for all present, which allows them to talk openly about the incident in a non-threatening way. Many debriefing-group members have difficulty discussing their personal feelings about the event but can participate in a discussion that focuses instead on the facts of the incident.

During the Thought Phase, participants are given the opportunity to express their immediate thoughts at the time of the critical incident. By encouraging expression of personal thoughts, this phase serves as a transitional stage between the impersonal facts surrounding the event to the more personal aspects of the event. The prevailing emotions of the members are likely to become evident during this phase, as individuals begin to respond to questions about their thoughts at the time of the event.

Emotions often reach their peak during the Reaction Phase of the debriefing as individuals are invited to address personal aspects of their experience. This phase ideally flows naturally from the previous phases and facilitators play a less active role. Anyone wishing to speak may do so and responses typically include crying, anger, expressions of guilt, and frustration. Personal comments, such as discussion of "the worst thing about the situation," what causes individuals the most pain, or whether there was a part they wish they could erase, all allow for individuals to vent about their experience, creating a cathartic emotional response in group members.

The Symptom Phase acts as another transitional phase, from a highly emotional level of processing back to a more cognitive level of understanding the event. Participants normalize each other's reactions by describing any cognitive, behavioural, emotional, or physical reactions that they are experiencing, or may have experienced, at the scene. Individuals are able to recognize that their reaction is not a sign of weakness or of vulnerability, but instead a normal reaction to the events described.

Flowing from the previous phase, the Teaching Phase allows the debriefing team the opportunity to acknowledge the symptoms described by the individuals, again reassuring them that their reactions are normal following the type of incident they experienced. The debriefers educate the individuals on each of the types of symptoms they are experiencing, and prepare the group for the potential development of other symptoms in the future. During this phase the debriefing team also spends time providing information on various stress-management strategies, such as relevant information about diet, exercise, relaxation, and talking to family or friends. As well, information is provided regarding using further use of the organization's EAP, or how to access other mental health practitioners in the community as an additional resource for those who may desire further help. This phase prepares individuals for the final stage of the debriefing by continuing to move the focus of the discussion away from the emotional content of earlier stages.

Finally the Re-entry Phase is used as an opportunity to clarify outstanding issues, answer questions, and also allow the participants to make final comments about their experience. Participants are encouraged to introduce anything new that they wish to discuss, review things they have learned and will be taking away from the debriefing, and ask questions about anything they feel may further help them bring closure to the debriefing. The responsibility of the debriefing team is to answer any questions, inform and reassure individuals, provide appropriate handouts or referrals to resources, and make summary comments of the debriefing to participants (Everly, Lating, & Mitchell, 2000).

Evidence-Based Practice

No matter what debriefing model is used, a number of key components must be present for CISD to be effective. These include psycho-education, mutual support, emotional release, and stress-management techniques (Mitchell & Bray, 1990; Regeher, 2001). Central to the success of debriefing is the fact that "humans respond in predictable ways to life-threatening emergencies, and that these responses are not in any way abnormal" (Kirk and Madden, 2003). There is evidence that short-term crisis intervention such as CISD can be as effective as long-term interventions, as long as they are well-structured and applied correctly (Mitchell, 1983; Robinson & Mitchell, 1993). Though CISD was not intended to be a "one-shot" intervention, separate from the other components of CISM (Every & Mitchell, 1997), crisis workers have found it necessary at times to apply the CISD process outside of the context of the full CISM framework. Additionally, CISD should be distinguished from "defusing," which is a process that occurs immediately following an incident, ideally within three to eight hours of a critical incident (Campfield & Hills, 2001). Shorter, unstructured debriefings, which encourage a brief discussion of the events, can result in a significant reduction in acute stress reactions. However, if a defusing is not achieved within twelve hours, a full formal debriefing within 72 hours of the incident is recommended (Kowalski, 1995).

Although the benefits associated with CISD can also be gained in individual debriefings, the ideal debriefing occurs with the group of individuals who shared the traumatic experience (Kirk & Madden, 2003). Miller (2001) points out that groups stimulate affiliation and social support, and that they are effective in connecting group members with community resources. Though debriefing groups are typically not intended to be therapy groups, it is recognized that in reality they have an important therapeutic impact. Clearly, the participants of the debriefing will relate best and offer each other support when they recognize that the other participants have similar feelings associated with their first-hand experience of the event.

In some instances, studies have discussed the benefits of having not only a professional but also a volunteer peer co-facilitator who is familiar with the details of the job situation and the organization. In the hospital, for example, a nurse familiar with the details of the job can work alongside a social worker skilled in psychological debriefing in order to assist emergency-room personnel who are treating victims of a tragic accident. Further, a peer volunteer who is not personally involved in delivering services to critically injured patients can provide increased empathy through first-hand knowledge of the positions of group members (Spitzer & Neely, 1992).

Social Workers and CISD

Many of the key principles and tools unique to social work practice make social workers particularly suitable to co-ordinate and lead debriefing teams.

Social workers as multidisciplinary team members are frequently involved in the education that is a critical component of CISD. In the debriefing process, the dissemination of information about normal responses to stress is essential in helping clients understand the range of symptoms they are experiencing. Social workers can also teach constructive and effective coping strategies to help clients manage stress responses. Another important aspect of CISD is to help identify individuals who may need further professional help following the debriefing: this is an essential part of social work discharge planning. Social work has a long history in the health-care field, though a somewhat shorter one in the general occupational assistance sector, of delivering crisis intervention services to victims and family members of tragic accidents and terminal illnesses. Spitzer and Neely (1992) suggest that the provision of social work counselling can extend beyond patient to patient-care staff, again demonstrating the benefits of social workers in debriefings of critical incidents. Extensive involvement in the education of patients and families, as well as in-service training for staff, indicates that these professionals are ideally suited to deliver critical debriefing services. In general, the profession of social work, through its involvement in the development of crisis-intervention counselling, has demonstrated its proficiency in helping clients manage crisis situations, as well as its suitability to conduct psychological debriefings.

Employee Assistance Programs

The appropriate use of CISD within a CISM framework can effectively address the reactions individuals experience following a traumatic event. Employee Assistance Programs (EAPs) that include services to address the stressful events impacting individuals provide a proven benefit to employees (Arthur, 2000; Spitzer & Neely, 1992). EAPs recognize the importance of resolving the effects of stress induced from overwhelming circumstances in both the working and non-working environment. Thus, EAPs that incorporate specific methods of addressing traumatic events experienced by employees at the workplace provide a tremendous additional benefit to employers as well. Assuming that successful debriefing alleviates immediate stress reactions and reduces the risk of developing serious post-traumatic stress symptoms, there are obvious benefits for any organization. Incorporating CISD and CISM into an organization's EAP leads to "an earlier return to duty by employees, a quicker return to former levels of efficiency and productivity, and reduced absenteeism and financial loss through workers' compensation claims." (Campfield & Hill, 2001).

Individuals in work settings who have been involved in debriefings have reported the positive effects they have experienced following their participation. For example, participants in a CISD program for hospital-based health-care personnel describe

> the relief associated with sharing individual emotional reactions to difficult situations, the increased awareness of the emotional and behavioural effects of stress on immediate colleagues, the heightened sense of being part of a professional health care team, and the increased likelihood that staff members will intervene individually and collectively when they identify negative stressors in their work (Spitzer & Burke, 1993).

Obviously there are very clear benefits for organizations that make available to their employees some form of critical-incident debriefing and CISM program.

Research

The nature of disasters and critical incidents make good-quality research difficult to design and implement. Research in the aftermath of trauma with survivors and affected individuals is extremely challenging given that the primary need is to help people cope with the immediate crises and not to study their responses to the counselling being provided. Mitchell's (1983) early findings did provide evidence that emergency-response workers who receive debriefing following exposure to severe situations recover more rapidly than those who do not receive debriefing, and also that fewer suffer from negative long-term emotional effects. Later research on CISD has further demonstrated the beneficial effects of critical-incident debriefing, which include a reduction in the number of reported post-traumatic stress symptoms, more prompt emotional recovery, and improved mental health. A meta-analysis of five previously published investigations found that the CISD model of psychological debriefing was an effective method of crisis intervention (Everly & Boyle, 1999). However, it is important to note that the therapeutic effects of debriefings are reduced as the application of CISD is delayed (Robinson & Mitchell, 1993; Raphael, Meldrum, & McFarlane, 1995).

Despite the research support for CISD as an effective intervention, research support has not been uniform. Although CISD was originally designed to be part of a broader CISM intervention and not used alone, van Emmerik et al (2002) evaluated CISD in a meta-analysis as a single-session debriefing after psychological trauma. CISD was administered within one month of a traumatic event to individuals and groups, and was reported to be ineffective in reducing symptoms of PTSD and other trauma-related symptoms. Seven studies were included in the final analysis, in which there were five CISD interventions, three non-CISD interventions, and six no-intervention controls. Single-session CISD was found to be less effective than non-CISD interventions and than no treatment at all. The authors point to several possible reasons for these findings, and suggest that CISD may interfere with the natural processing of a traumatic experience and that individuals may become further sensitized to reminders of the trauma. Another possibility is that CSID might inadvertently cause the client to refrain from discussing their experience with family and friends, thus bypassing a natural system of support. There was also concern that the process of debriefing might cause individuals to see themselves as more medically damaged than they normally would. They suggested that further research look at the benefits of targeting at-risk individuals rather than treating all affected individuals in a group debriefing (van Emmerik et al 2002).

The Cochrane Review (Rose, Bisson, & Wessely 2004) also found no current evidence that single-session individual psychological *debriefing* is a useful treatment for the prevention of PTSD after traumatic incidents. They analyzed 11 relevant studies and reported that those most at risk for developing PTSD and other psychological outcomes are unlikely to be helped by a single session of CISD. They also found CISD had no effect on individuals with symptoms of anxiety and depression following a traumatic event. They raised the concern that some individuals may be negatively affected by a single CISD session, and concluded that "At present the routine use of single session individual debriefing in the aftermath of individual trauma cannot be recommended in either military or civilian life" (Rose et al, 2004). The authors acknowledge that they could not comment on the use of group debriefing, debriefing after mass traumas, or on the debriefing of children because of insufficient data on these issues. It is possible that the intervention might have been too short to allow for the emotional processing of trauma material, possibly re-traumatizing the individual and exacerbating their symptoms. Similarly they consider the possibility that more time is required between the trauma event and its treatment, to allow a natural de-escalation in the individual's response before it is re-examined in a debriefing session. They also note there is some evidence to show that individuals who have a strong shame reaction to the trauma are more at risk of trauma-related disorders. It suggests that these individuals might form an interesting subgroup for further research. A further consideration emanating from these studies is whether in fact there has been such a broad cultural acceptance of debriefing following trauma that it renders a formal debriefing intervention unnecessary. The argument is that there is sufficient general awareness of "psychological first aid" such that debriefing occurs anyway and thus reduces the possibility of demonstrating any effects from a formal treatment. The authors wonder whether debriefing techniques might be better aimed at managing a traumatic incident rather than mitigating traumatic symptoms—and believes that the aims of treatment need to be re-considered. They note that further research is of particular urgency in the efficacy of debriefing in emergency workers, group debriefing, and debriefing after mass disasters (Rose et al, 2004).

Evidence-based practice requires research support for the development of interventions, which are effective in dealing with exposure to traumatic events. Research must examine whether in fact psychological debriefing is as safe and useful as intuitive processes suggest. Nonetheless, it would be unwise to ignore some earlier positive findings about CISD or to abandon debriefing as a potentially useful intervention. Further trials of debriefing with different groups under various conditions are needed in order to identify the particular elements that are important in helping people overcome the effects of traumatic exposure, particularly within EAP environments. Everly, Flannery, and Mitchell (2000) have noted the importance of conducting research on the many facets of the CISM model and suggest that future guidelines and policies be "increasingly empirically driven" to ensure that all clients exposed to critical incidents receive evidence-based intervention.

Endnotes

1. Spitzer & Neely, 1992; Spitzer & Burke, 1993; Everly, Lating, & Mitchell, 2000; Regeher, 2001.
2. For a more detailed discussion of crisis theory please refer to chapter 10.

References

Arthur, A.R. (2000). Employee Assistance Programmes: The emperor's new clothes of stress management? *British Journal of Guidance and Counselling* 28(4), 549–560.

Bell, J. (1995). Traumatic event debriefing: Service delivery designs and the role of social work. *Social Work* 40, 36–44.

Campfield, K. M. and Hills, A.M. (2001). Effect of timing of critical incident stress debriefing (CISD) on posttraumatic symptoms. *Journal of Traumatic Stress* 14, 327–340.

Conroy, R.J. (1990, February). Critical incident stress debriefing. *FBI Law Enforcement Bulletin* 20–22.

Everly, G.S. (1990). *A clinical guide to the treatment of the human stress response*. New York: Plenum Press.

Everly, G.S. (1999). A primer on critical incident stress management: What's really in a name. *International Journal of Emergency Mental Health* 1(2), 76–78.

Everly, G.S. Jr. & Boyle S.H. (1999). Critical incident stress debriefing (CISD): A meta-analysis. *International Journal of Emergency Mental Health* 1(3), 165–168.

Everly, G.S., Boyle, S.H. & Lating, J.M. (1999). The effectiveness of psychological debriefing with vicarious trauma: A meta-analysis. *Stress Medicine* 15, 229–233.

Everly, G.S. & Mitchell, J.T. (1997). *Critical incident stress management (CISM): A new era and standard of care in crisis intervention.* Ellicott City, MD: Chevron.

Everly, G.S. & Mitchell, J.T. (1999). *Critical incident stress management (CISM): A new era and standard of care in crisis intervention* (2nd edn). Ellicott City, MD: Chevron.

Everly, G.S., Flannery, R.B., & Mitchell, J.T. (2000). Critical incident stress management (CISM): A review of the literature. *Aggression and Violent Behaviour* 5(1), 23–40.

Everly, G.S., Lating, J.M., & Mitchell, J.T. (2000). Innovations in group crisis intervention. In Roberts, A.R. (ed.), *Crisis intervention handbook assessment, treatment and research* (2nd edn.). Ellicott City, MD: International Critical Incident Stress Foundation.

Everly, G.S. & Mitchell, J.T. (2000). *Critical stress management: Advanced group crisis interventions: A workbook.* Ellicott City, MD: International Critical Incident Stress Foundation.

Gist, R. & Lubin, B. (1989). *Psychosocial aspects of disaster.* New York: John Wiley & Sons.

Kirk, A.B. & Madden, L.L. (2003). Trauma-related critical incident debriefing for adolescents. *Child and Adolescent Social Work Journal* 20, 123–134.

Kowalski, K.M. (1995). A human component to consider in your emergency management plans: The critical incident stress factor. *Safety Science* 20, 115–123.

McFarlane, A.C. & Yehuda, R. (1996). Resilience, vulnerability and the course of postraumatic reactions. In B.A. van der Kolk, A.C. McFarlane, & L. Weisaeth (eds), *Traumatic stress: The effects of overwhelming experience on mind, body, and society.* New York: The Guilford Press.

Miller, J. (2001). The use of debriefing in schools. *Smith College in Social Work* 71, 259–272.

Mitchell, J.T. (1983). When disaster strikes. The critical incident stress debriefing process. *Journal of Emergency Medical Services* 8(1), 36–39.

Mitchell, J.T. & Bray, G. (1990). *Emergency services stress: Guidelines for preserving the health and careers of emergency services personnel.* Englewood Cliffs, NJ: Prentice Hall.

Mitchell, J.T. & Everly, G. (1993). *Critical incident stress debriefings*. Ellicott City, MD: Chevron.

Raphael, B. (1986). *When disaster strikes: A handbook for caring professionals*. London: Unwin Hyman.

Raphael, B. Meldrum, L., & McFarlane, A. (1995). Does debriefing after psychological trauma work? *British Medical Journal*. 310, 1479–1480.

Rapoport, L. (1967). Crisis-oriented short-term casework. *Social Service Review* 41, 31–43.

Regeher, C. (2001). Crisis debriefing groups for emergency responders: Reviewing the evidence. *Brief Treatment and Crisis Intervention* 1, 87–100.

Robinson, R.C. & Mitchell, J.T. (1993). Evaluation of psychological debriefings. *Journal of Traumatic Stress* 6, 367–382.

Rose, S. & Bisson, J. (1998). Brief early psychological interventions following trauma: A systematic review of the literature. *Journal of Traumatic Stress* 11, 697–710.

Rose, S., Wessley, S., & Bisson, J. (2002). Psychological debriefing for preventing post traumatic stress disorder (PTSD). Cochrane Database of Systemic Reviews.

Spitzer, W. & Burke, L.A (1993). Critical incident stress debriefing program for hospital-based health care personnel. *Health & Social Work* 18(2), 149–156.

Spitzer, W. & Neely, K. (1992). Critical incident stress: The role of hospital-based social work in developing a statewide intervention system for first-responders delivering emergency services. *Social Work in Health Care* 18, 39–58.

Van Emmerik, A.A., Kamphuis, J.H., Hulsbosch, A.M., & Emmelkamp P.M. (2002). Single session debriefing after psychological trauma: a meta-analysis. *Lancet* 7, 360(9335), 766–771.

van der Kolk, B. (1987). *Psychological trauma*. Washington, D.C.: American Psychiatric Press.

12

Brief Counselling
in Employee Assistance

Wayne Skinner

Introduction

There is a particularly close relationship between Employee Assistance Programming (EAP) and Brief Treatment/Therapy (BT). If Brief Treatment did not exist, EAP might well have had to invent it. Otherwise, the clinical service EAP providers offer might well be reduced to assessment and referral. Instead, Brief Treatment allows EAP practitioners a powerful medium for working with clients within the limited context of EAP work, with a reasonable expectation that they can be helpful to the individuals who seek help from them. This means that the EAP counsellor can capably address a broad range of human problems, from mild to moderate to severe. Brief Treatment also enhances the options on which a prospective mental-health or social-service consumer has to draw. The one requirement of potential clients is that they or their family members be employed by a company that offers this service as a benefit to its employees.

Brief Treatment also makes EAP services an additionally attractive element in a company's employee benefits package, as EAP enhances the wellness and productivity of a workforce in which it usually has made a significant investment. It should be noted that employers offer these services not necessarily because of fundamentally altruistic reasons; rather, it is as a means of protecting the investment they have made in the human capital that they employ. At the same time, however, it should also be acknowledged that users of these services tend to report high rates of satisfaction, and perceive advantages to using these services above those available in the public sector. Usually there is quick access to EAP services, and EAP service providers are highly motivated to make sure that the consumer is satisfied with the assistance provided.

169

EAP provides a wide range of services, including counselling and therapy for psychosocial issues ranging from work stress to marital conflict to trauma, depression, and bereavement. This brief essay can only accomplish a few modest tasks, not unlike BT itself. First, I would like to examine the strong evidence base for BT. Then, I will advance the argument that method and approach are not as important in BT as the interpersonal factors that construct the therapeutic relationship between client and helper. BT tends to be a dynamic, active process that encourages a partnership between client and helper. This helps us construct the helping project in BT in ways that do not devolve into narrow notions of pathology and illness, but rather reinforce the possibility of change, renewal, and transformation within the framework of the client as active agent and partner in the helping enterprise. This allows us to move away from the typical comparisons of schools and ideologies of BT, and helps us see BT as a set of deliberate and negotiated human processes between client and helper, which involves identifying concerns, needs, and problems, and working towards goals, desires and solutions. At the same time, this event, even if built on confidentiality and privacy, does not occur in isolation, but inheres in a broader surround of life issues that include the power relations and politics of everyday life, the play of circumstance, and the human realities of mutability and finitude.

Once we have made the case for BT in this way, it will be important to turn the coin over and undertake another critique, again all too brief, this time of the limits and pitfalls and problematics of this approach to care. As surely as there is a strong case to be made for Brief Treatment in EAP practice, so are there cautions and red flags that need to be recognized. All of this is offered in the belief that knowledge and practice are both "arguable" domains of human activity, that they should be held up, inspected, made to explain themselves, and used as springboards for better concepts and responses to human problems, which is the humanistic foundation that should underlie all of our efforts as helpers, whatever our disciplinary stripe and ideological persuasion.

The Case for Brief Treatment: Reviewing the Evidence

Much of the history of psychotherapy research is a celebration of the "null hypothesis," the conclusion that researchers have most often come to when they have compared one form of therapy to another. More often than not, the report is that when people are randomly assigned to one of two conditions, they do equally as well in either situation. This has meant that in a great many studies interventions of shorter duration were as effective as longer-term interventions. This includes treatments as brief as one session compared to as much as therapy as a client can get his or her hands on (Orford & Edwards, 1997). So the vast archive that now exists on psychotherapy research looks very favourably upon Brief Treatment.

However, one can have some reservations about the research methodology used in much of this research. Such research usually requires that clients receive comprehensive assessments and be actively followed up for months and even years to measure outcome. Though there is a tendency to make bald comparisons between treatments of short and extended duration, it is important to note that the contacts such research requires erode the argument that a single session does the trick as well as extended treatment. In both conditions in such research the client is involved in an apparatus of intervention that involves thorough assessment and systematic follow-up. Even if the research events are not intentionally therapeutic, the processes they put clients through, especially if they are done with respect and sensitivity, have therapeutic effects. To truly evaluate Brief Treatment, one would need a method of research that did not exceed the intervention in the duration and intensity of its involvement.

This point might seem unnecessary to some, but it is as important for clinicians to interrogate the logic and method of research as it is for clinical theory and practice to be open to similar interrogation by researchers. In fact, it allows one to note that most of the research on which best-practice evidence is based takes place with very narrowly defined client populations. They tend to be deliberately chosen because their "lack of complexity" makes them more straightforward subjects of research and follow-up. While the results may possess strong internal validity, the confidence with which findings can be applied to much more diverse and complex "real-world" populations is regrettably low. The need to question the "ecological-validity" of research, and to resist the tendency for false generalizability, is important in building what could be called "really useful knowledge" on which to inform clinical practice. Brief Treatment research suffers from this deficiency as much as any domain of psychotherapy research.

With those two caveats noted, the convergent evidence supporting Brief Treatment is nonetheless very strong and persuasive. Asay and Lambert (1999), after conducting a meta-analysis of six decades of psychotherapy, conclude that there is little to doubt: "Therapy is effective. Treated patients fare much better than the untreated" (24). They add to that claim the observation that the path to positive change is not long for most people, and that the benefits are sustained. The durability of Brief Treatment and other psychosocial interventions is an important consideration, one often forgotten today in the strong bias towards pharmacotherapies as panacea for most human problems. Drug therapies produce effects that last as long as the drug action. Psychotherapies confer extended benefits. In addition, we are discovering that withdrawing and tapering from many drugs can be challenging and difficult, as we have discovered with many pharmaceuticals that were initially compelling, but are now being held up for more balanced appraisal. Two decades ago, this was being done with benzodiazepines; today we are doing it with SSRIs such as Prozac and Paxil. Asay and Lambert (1999) conclude, "That psychotherapy is, in general, effective, efficient, and lasting has been empirically supported time and again" (28).

A question that follows from that overall conclusion is: what then works best for what kinds of people with what kinds of problem? This question has recurrently led researchers in a circle back to the null hypothesis. The most eloquent example of this happens to be the most expensive and elaborate psychotherapy trial ever undertaken. Project MATCH (Matching Alcoholism Treatment To Client Heterogeneity) cost US$ 27 million. It compared three interventions—cognitive behavioural therapy (CBT), motivational enhancement therapy (MET), and Twelve-Step Facilitation (TSF). Each therapy was conducted over 12 weeks, after a comprehensive evaluation, and followed by three years of follow-up. CBT and TSF saw clients weekly, while MET involved only four sessions over the 12 weeks. This study, which involved over 1,600 participants, was intended to determine the key client characteristics that would predict outcomes in very different treatments. The first findings of the study were published in 1997: "Project MATCH is the largest, statistically most powerful, psychotherapy trial ever conducted. The limited findings ... challenge the existing view that attribute by treatment matching is a key to improved treatment effectiveness .... Except for psychiatric severity, there is no convincing evidence of major matching effects. Matching ... did not enhance treatment effectiveness" (Project MATCH, 1977, p. 25).

As demoralizing as this must have been for the researchers, there was a finding that is ultimately more important: clients in each of the conditions had very positive outcomes—drinking days dropped from over 80 percent to less than 20 percent, and saw very little deterioration over three years of follow-up. These interventions were carefully developed and manualized, with counsellors trained in the method and all sessions taped to ensure fidelity to the treatment model. This recent study is the most eloquent reiteration of decades of research that recommends brief treatments, but not any particular form or method of treatment.

What are the implications of these finding for Brief Treatment? First of all, from an effectiveness perspective, Brief Treatment could be considered the intervention of first resort for many human problems. Asay and Lambert (1999) through their meta-analyses found that about half of clients in psychotherapy showed significant change in five to ten sessions of therapy. Extending the number to 26 sessions or six months increased the number from 50 percent to 75 percent. Their advice is that "therapists organize their work to optimize outcomes within a few sessions" (42). How then to do that? That is the topic to which we will now turn.

Practicing Brief Treatment

There are a dizzying number of brief therapies that have been described and operationalized by clinicians.[1] Today we might first think of cognitive behaviour therapy, solution-focused therapy, strategic-interactional therapies, brief couple and family therapies, brief group psychotherapies, and humanistic therapies such as gestalt. However, there are brief variations of therapies that are stereotypically very extended—psychodynamic therapies, including psychoanalysis. However, if we are instructed by the earlier discussion, this array of methods is both to be expected, and not to be respected, as the primary locus of an effective understanding of what Brief Treatment is all about and how it works.

The argument supported by what we know about counselling and therapy is that the most important variable is the therapeutic relationship. This point has been well argued by numerous theorists since Carl Rogers (1953). Lambert (1992) concluded after a comprehensive cultural review of the psychotherapy literature that the therapeutic relationship accounted for 30 percent of the variance in treatment outcome. Method or approach only had half the power (15 percent) in determining outcome, as did expectancy, a critical variable not to be forgotten or minimized. These three factors represent the three cards a counsellor has to play in the helping process. Importantly, Lambert found that 40 percent of the factors affecting treatment outcome belonged to the client. The more social support, or social capital, as compellingly conceptualized by Bourdieu (1993), the more likely the outcome would be positive (Bourdieu & Wacquant, 1995). Along with the other forms of capital, economic and cultural, social capital is a potent determinant of the likelihood of developing the kinds of problems that draw people to psychotherapy, and the odds that they will get a successful outcome. However, we know that these factors, while powerful, do not over-determine outcomes. Psychological and biological factors also play essential roles in shaping the strengths and disadvantages that clients bring with them to the counselling context. The need to take a comprehensive holistic approach to understanding and working with a client's concerns is increasingly important, not just for reasons of clinical efficacy, but also for issues related to liability and professional standards (this will be further discussed below).

Using this schema of four key domains, on one hand, client factors, and on the other hand, the therapeutic relationship, expectancy, and method/ technique, one sees that the most important factor the EAP provider can influence is the counselling alliance, by being able to engage and motivate the client. The next most important function is to enhance the client's hope that the process will be helpful, followed by applying techniques and methods that lead to sustainable change.

Brief Treatment usually involves the deliberate and active use of the EAP counsellor's ability to establish a strong working relationship with the client and to use it to determine, through dialogue and negotiation with the client, what the focus of the work should be. I will look at the helping process by describing six essential activities: engagement, understanding, planning, taking action, reviewing process, and ending.

i) Engagement
    Where the formal view would be that the first thing a counsellor should undertake is assessment, I would counter that firstly, and continuing throughout, the primary therapeutic task is engagement. This is the process of connecting with the client in ways that lead to the client's belief that they are with someone who is interested in them, who wants to understand their issues and concerns, hopes and goals, and who will be helpful and committed to working with them to find effective responses and solutions to their problems. The primary way that engagement is achieved is through active listening, which involves a tuneful understanding of what client is saying, verbally and nonverbally. It requires the client's acknowledgement to be accomplished, rather than the counsellor's self-satisfied conclusion that they are doing a fine job. The client does this by feedback, which affirms that they experience the helper as being in tune with them and that the unfolding events in the counselling process are addressing the client's needs and goals. This task of engagement continues throughout the helping process, and the transition to different phases of work can raise challenges to engagement that must be skillfully addressed. For example, going from talking about a concern to taking action puts the relationship and the process on a different footing.

ii) Understanding
    The second phase in Brief Treatment is assessment, which can also be conceptualized as "understanding." "Understanding" represents

the emerging knowledge that the helper has of the client, and also of the collaborative knowledge that is produced and held in common by both participants in the process. The EAP counsellor facilitates this by using the particular skills that come from the model of care in which he or she is working. Understanding requires the counsellor to be tunefully aware of the client in the client's own terms, but then organizing this awareness through a lens that is usually the product of the helper's approach to working: the theories, concepts, and experience that they have to draw upon. This has to pass the test of leading to action: is the client at least willing to try a new or altered behaviour with some enthusiasm? Or, better yet, is the client excited and animated, moving from a preoccupation with the problem to a focus on the solution? One way this may be accomplished is through a formal process of assessment and diagnosis, in which a formal identity is given to the client's problems. Indeed, one of the functions of such formal processes is to give a name to the client's problems and, based on that, to recommend a prescribed course of action. To the degree that the client is agreeable to the counsellor's expert reading of the problem and its solution, there is an enhanced likelihood that the intervention will work. However, such formal procedures are not the only way to come to an understanding of what is wrong, what is needed, and how to proceed. Some therapies indeed are effective because they actively resist conforming to such orthodox procedures (Haley, 1974; Cade & O'Hanlon, 1993).

iii) Planning
When the client and worker have developed a shared understanding of what the issue is, and what needs to be done about it, the next step becomes making a plan of action. What is to be done? By whom? When? For how long? It tends to be helpful to bring as much specificity as possible to understanding what is wrong and what to do about it. The more the focus of the work of Brief Treatment can be particularized, the easier it should be to work out action steps and sequences. As that becomes clearer, the stage is set for action.

The primary ethic in Brief Treatment is working with the client as a partner and collaborator in a process of change, or more accurately, seeing the EAP counsellor as a resource and a guide to the client, who is seeking to solve a problem or make a change. The task of planning can be a fairly straightforward negotiation, or it can be a process that is led by either partner in the process. Sometimes the counsellor might step back and let the client try it his or her way. Sometimes the client might be confused and perplexed and seeking guidance from the EAP counsellor. One way of finding out the client's expectation of the counsellor is to ask, how much direction do you want me to take at this point in our work? Do you want me to offer advice that you will try out? Or would you rather tell me what you want to do and use me as a resource in making your plans? Clients usually give good feedback about this, and even when the counsellor is playing a directive role, it is at the client's request (Sobell, Sobell, Bogardis, & Skinner, 1992).

iv) Taking Action

If the work to this point can be characterized as connecting, exploring, and talking about options, this phase involves the doing. The skills required to take action are more than the ability to understand a problem and plan a solution. In many approaches in Brief Treatment, it is not uncommon for the EAP counsellor to be willing to work actively as a coach, helping the client with the practical skills that are often essential for successful change, while building the client's self-efficacy. A key aspect of this phase is to make sure that the tasks are realistically challenging, without overwhelming the client, so that the client achieves them with a strong sense of accomplishment.

v) Reviewing Progress

As things proceed, it is important to identify how well goals are being met. Even if they are met, that is not the measure of success. Instead, that is determined by the client's feedback about whether the new state is more desirable than the previous one, and worth working to maintain. More often than not the process of working on this causes goals and targets to change. The engaged EAP counsellor is always alert to taking the measure of this and applying a realistic approach to the helping process, picking up the pace, slowing it down, suggesting a change in focus as events indicate.

vi) Ending

Endings are usually difficult tasks for people, especially if the experience of which they have been part has been positive and successful. It is important for the helper to normalize this stage, and to legitimize the client's particular feelings. One of the things a client in counselling should experience is a good ending, one that has been performed to a high level by the EAP counsellor, and hopefully by the client as well. At the same time that an episode of care and of work is concluding, the client needs to know if the door is open for return, and what the options are if they need to seek help again.

Summary

Six essential activities may seem like an ambitious structure to impose on brief therapy, but in fact all of these components of the brief counselling process could be played out in even a single session. Indeed, it can be helpful to try to give each session this shape, as a way of bringing organization and direction to the process. Some approaches to Brief Treatment have very discrete boundaries around the phases in the process (Antonuccio, Lewinsohn, Piasecki, & Ferguson 2000), while in other approaches the distinction between the phases blurs, so that even in the first session, a plan is contracted and client and counsellor are in the action stage.

The Role of the EAP Counsellor in Brief Treatment

The overview constructed suggests that the method may in fact be more important to the worker than to the client. The benefits that this method confers are consequent more to the confidence it gives the worker and the order it brings to the helping project. In most cases any one method rarely has inherent advantages over another: this has been the findings of many studies, which maintain that of all of the interventions under consideration are effective, without finding advantage in any particular approach.

Generally, the role of the counsellor in Brief Treatment is an active one. Even when the EAP counsellor is taking a non-directive approach, there is a high level of intentionality in the way the counsellor shapes the interactive process and the direction it takes. What Jay Haley (1973) says of strategic therapy can be said more generally of Brief Treatment: it is the task of the counsellor to identify solvable problems, to work with the client to set goals, to design interventions that achieve these goals, and to explore the responses to these interventions.

The Role of the EAP Client in Brief Treatment

Even when the worker is confident and convinced, it is not uncommon for a client to feel ambivalent and reluctant. In many ways, it is the client's job to be like that, just as it is ours to help the client to stay hopeful and committed. It may be the outcome about which the client feels ambivalent, although more often than not, the client has a strong identification with the desired outcome. The client is more likely to be ambivalent in their belief about the likelihood of achieving the goal, or of what might have to change in order to achieve the change they desire. If the EAP counsellor expects the client to be struggling with the need to change, or with their confidence that they can effect change, it is much easier to be not just empathically supportive, but also more effective in helping the client to move forward.

Prochaska and DiClimente (1984) describe the process of change as consisting of phases. By being able to locate where the client is in that process, and by understanding the key challenges the client has to face if they are going to move to the next phase, the counsellor can play an active and deliberate role in bringing this about. The initial stage is "Precontemplation": the client is not thinking about the need to change. The task of the counsellor here is to persuade the client to perceive that there might be some aspects of the client's behaviour or situation that are problematic. In the next stage, "Contemplation," the client becomes aware that there are some good and some not-so-good aspects to a behaviour or a situation. They can see the two sides to the behaviour. However, on balance they still have not resolved to experiment with change. "Preparation," the third stage, is characterized by the client making statements about imminent change and making plans to effect change. The EAP counsellor's job here is to reinforce the merits of positive change and validate the client's ability to make change. This leads to the "Action" stage, in which the client is working to make the change happen. The counsellor's role here can be help the client learn and apply the skills needed to make the change stick, and to affirm the client's ability to make intentional change in their lives. This stage, as it succeeds, leads to "Maintenance." No longer is the work of change a preoccupation, but the client is still at risk of relapse. The EAP counsellor can help the client by preparing them for high-risk situations, anticipating challenges, and developing relapse-prevention strategies. All the way along, there is a risk of relapse, of the client abandoning their goals, and falling back into the problematic behaviour or situation they were trying to escape. The merits of this approach are significant. They include giving the counsellor a means of assessing the client's stage, and using appropriate techniques of engagement. The Stages of Change Model helps both client and worker see change as a process. Therapy becomes the challenge of aligning counselling resources to the client's larger processes of change. When this is done effectively, change can be accomplished more successfully. It also suggests that counsellors might go about doing work in ways that could delay, oppose, or undermine the client's potential for constructive, intentional change.

Challenges in Brief Treatment

Increasingly, the field of counselling and therapy is being professionalized. In addition, we live in a culture that is becoming increasing litigious. Consumers expect positive results, and when these do not eventuate, they may seek remedy through civil suit or through complaints to professional bodies. These are actually progressive developments in that they increase professional accountability and client empowerment, and they have a shaping effect on clinical practice that has a strong impact on Brief Treatment and Therapy. The need to be professionally accountable is often manifest in a requirement that the counsellor conduct a thorough and comprehensive assessment of the client that is documented in detail. In BT it is expected that clients can present their concerns and goals quite directly, and that that is sufficient for getting down to work with them. An added emphasis on comprehensive assessment and thorough documentation inhibits the ability of the EAP counsellor to quickly move to action mode, or to take the client at the explicit level in which they present.

Added to that, there are growing expectations that clinicians will assess risk in the client, both to self-harm and to violence towards others. It could be that the requirement to ensure that standard procedures were used to determine the client's risk could interfere with BT approaches that are reliably effective and responsive to the needs of many clients who are ready to take action towards positive change. EAP providers are particularly sensitive to their own risks and liabilities, and have introduced more structured assessment requirements. These have the effect of reshaping the work that is undertaken in EAP and the way time is used. Given that the temporal boundaries are quite tightly drawn, the worker who is required to work in a manner that is largely preoccupied with documentation and risk-avoidance could undermine the goals and values of BT. It could be that EAP turns towards the assessment and referral functions, and leaves too little to the direct negotiation of worker and client. Instead a procedural and documentary superstructure overtakes the great opportunities to work actively and immediately with clients on solvable problems on a direct-action basis. Certainly the recent moves to structure and standardize the documentary requirements in EAP work do have a shaping effect on the ways counsellors can use the limited time they have with their clients. The direction of these developments is away from client-centered processes, and towards ensuring that the professional and legal liabilities of the counsellor and the agency are protected by a veil of documentation.

Nonetheless, these changes do not subvert EAP services in a fatal way. They should encourage counsellors to reflect on the ways in which they work with clients, and the ways they can preserve the more fundamental ethic of being client-centered, and directing resources to people with problems rather than enacting subtle procedures of social control and surveillance. They do remind us that the relationship that is enjoined when a client and a counsellor sit down together is not merely a dyadic one. It involves a third party (the payer), as well as a fourth (the EAP provider); and surrounding them are the "others"—the collaterals of the client and a very diverse social audience with its own beliefs about how psychosocial problems ought to be viewed and treated. Critical reflection and dialogue on this dynamic can form an essential basis for EAP professionals to construct their clinical practice and their professional roles in creating well workers and well workplaces.

Endnotes
1. Hersen & Biaggio, 2000; Winston & Winston, 2002; Cade & O'Hanlon, 1993; Hubble, Miller, & Duncan, 1999.

References

Antonuccio, D.O., Lewinsohn, P.M., Piasecki, M., & Ferguson, R. (2000). Major depressive episode. In M. Hersen & M. Biaggio (eds.), *Effective brief therapies: A clinician's guide*. San Diego: Academic Press.

Asay, T.P. & Lambert, M.J. (1999). The empirical case for the common factors in therapy: Quantitative findings. In M.A. Hubble, B.L. Duncan, & S.D. Miller (eds.), *The heart and soul of change: What works in therapy*. Washington: American Psychological Association.

Beck, A.T. (1976). *Cognitive therapy and the emotional disorders*. New York: International Universities Press.

Bourdieu, P., Parkhurst Ferguson, P., Emanuel, S., Johnson, J., Waryn, S.T., & Acardo, A. (1993). *The weight of the world: Social suffering in contemporary society*. Stanford: Stanford University Press.

Bourdieu P. & Wacquant, L. (1992). *An invitation to reflexive sociology*. Chicago: University of Chicago Press.

Cade, B. & O'Hanlon, W.H. (1993). *A brief guide to brief therapy*. New York: W.W. Norton.

De Shazer, S. (1992). *Putting difference to work*. New York: W.W. Norton.

Haley, J. (1973). *Uncommon therapy: Psychiatric techniques of Milton Erickson, M.D.* New York: W.W. Norton.

Hersen, M. & Biaggio, M. (eds.). (2000). *Effective brief therapies: A clinician's guide*. San Diego, CA: Academic Press.

Hubble, M.A., Duncan, B.L., & Miller, S.D. (eds.). (1999). *The heart and soul of change: What works in therapy*. Washington, DC: American Psychological Association.

Janis, I.L. (1983). *Short-term counselling: Guidelines based on recent research*. New Haven: Yale University Press.

Johnson, L.D. (1995). *Psychotherapy in the age of accountability*. New York: W.W. Norton.

Lambert, M.J. (1992). Implications of outcome research for psychotherapy integration. In J.C. Norcross & M.R. Goldstein (eds.), *Handbook of psychotherapy integration*. New York: Basic Books.

Miller, W.R. & Rollnick, S. (2002). *Motivational interviewing: Preparing people for change* (2nd edn). New York: Guilford Press.

Miller, S.D. & Berg I.K. (1995). *The miracle method: A radically new approach to problem drinking.* New York: Norton.

Orford, J. & Edwards, G. (1997). *Alcoholism: A comparison of treatment and advice, with a study of the influence of marriage.* Oxford: Oxford University Press.

Project MATCH Research Group. (1997). Matching alcoholism treatments to client heterogeneity: Project MATCH post-treatment outcomes. *Journal of Studies in Alcohol* 59, 631–639.

Prochaska, J. & DiClemente, C. (1984). *The transtheoretical model: Crossing traditional boundaries of therapy.* Homewood, IL.: Dow Jones/Irwin.

Rogers C. (1951). *Client-Centered therapy.* Boston: Houghton-Mifflin.

Sobell, L., Sobell, M., Bogardis, J., Leo, G.I., & Skinner, W. (1992). Problem drinkers' perceptions of whether treatment goals should be self-selected or therapist-selected. *Behavior Therapy* 23, 43–52.

Strupp, H.H. & Binder, J.L. (1984). *Psychotherapy in a new key: A guide to time-limited psychotherapy.* New York: Basic Books.

Winston, A. & Winston, B. (2002). *Handbook of integrated short-term psychotherapy.* Washington, DC: American Psychiatric Press.

13

Brief Treatment for Employees with Low-to-Moderate Alcohol Dependence:
A Guided Self-Change Approach

Marilyn Herie

Introduction

Brief Treatment has been defined variously in the literature, but is generally taken to mean community-based, as opposed to residential, interventions of 12 or fewer sessions. There is considerable research evidence for the efficacy of brief, secondary interventions for individuals with alcohol and other drug problems (Moyer et al., 2002; Dunn, Deroo, and Rivara, 2001). In addition, brief outpatient interventions have been found to have comparable outcomes with more intensive treatment approaches (Heather, 2002; Martin, Koski-Jannes, & Weber, 1998; Babor, 1994). For example, a recent study examining one- and eight-year drinking outcomes for individuals entering treatment for the first time found that individuals receiving Brief Treatment of eight or fewer sessions (or less intensive treatment of longer duration, entailing a few sessions spaced over many weeks or months), fared better at one- and eight-year follow-up than did an untreated control group (Moos & Moos, 2003). The authors also found that more intensive residential treatment was not associated with better outcomes. Thus, even very brief treatment models have been demonstrated to have an impact of lasting duration on individuals' alcohol and other drug use.

Of course, brief, outpatient treatment is not suitable for all clients. Addictive behaviour can be regarded as falling along a continuum of severity, anchored by mild levels of dependence at one end, and more severe, chronic dependence at the other. In addition, it is possible to conceptualize addiction interventions as falling along the same continuum, with "natural recovery," recovery without intervention, self-help, and brief treatments at one end, and more intensive day-treatment and residential programs at the other. Figure 13.1 illustrates how a range of treatment options fits with the continuum of severity.

Figure 13.1: Continuum of services for alcohol treatment

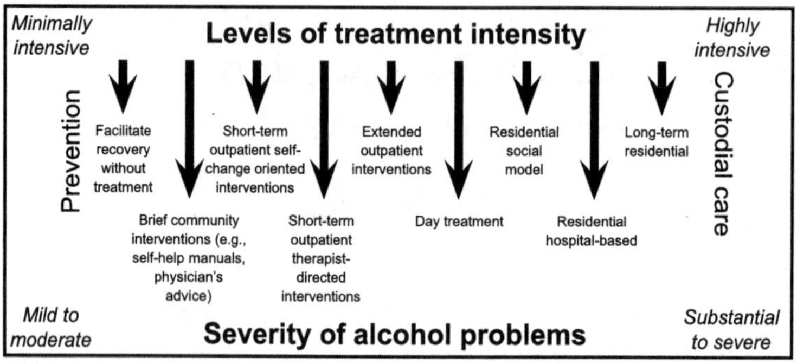

Adapted from: Centre for Addiction and Mental Health (CAMH), 1998a.

Figure 13.1 illustrates the importance of matching treatment interventions to the particular needs of clients. In this view, treatment spaces in intensive residential programs should be reserved for those who need them most, i.e., people with severe levels of alcohol or other drug dependence. The notion of "stepped care," which suggests that people start with the least intrusive level of treatment, fits with generally accepted medical practice. Using a stepped-care approach, individuals are matched to an appropriate level of treatment, treatment response is carefully monitored, and the intensity of treatment can be "stepped up" as needed. The validity of this approach has been buttressed by the large body of treatment-outcome research supporting the efficacy of brief, outpatient interventions, summarized in Health Canada's *Best Practices in Addiction Treatment* document (www.hc-sc.gc.ca/hecs-sesc/cds/pdf/best_pract.pdf).

The Guided Self-Change (GSC) approach discussed in this chapter provides an example of a research-based, brief-treatment model for individuals with mild to moderate levels of alcohol and other drug dependence (Sobell & Sobell, 1998; 1996; CAMH, 1998a; CAMH, 1998b), and has been adapted for use in community settings through field tests with counsellors from across Ontario, Canada (Martin et al., 1998).

Overview of the Guilded Self-Change Approach

The Guided Self-Change protocol entails four structured treatment sessions lasting approximately one hour each, which are designed to assist clients in mobilizing their internal resources to achieve abstinence or reduced-drinking goals. Unlike other community-based interventions designed for more severely dependent clients, the GSC approach does not teach coping skills; rather, the goal in treatment is to assist individuals in applying the problem-solving and coping strategies used in other life areas to resolving her current pattern of problem drinking. Thus, GSC can be viewed as a general problem-solving approach where, by the end of the treatment sessions, the client has become his or her own therapist.

GSC draws on a variety of theoretical frameworks and models, including cognitive-behavioural approaches,[1] motivational interviewing,[2] stages of change theory,[3] solution-focused therapy,[4] and research into natural recovery from alcohol problems.[5]

Each of the five GSC sessions is designed to build on the last, so that individuals progress from identifying and evaluating reasons for changing their drinking behaviour, to identifying situations that trigger problem-drinking episodes, to formulating plans for action and putting these into practice. Weekly readings and homework exercises reinforce the session content, and are designed to enhance motivation and provide opportunities to practice new strategies and behaviours.

It is important to emphasize that people with less severe alcohol problems differ in a number of ways from those with more severe levels of dependence. Individuals with low to moderate levels of dependence tend to have shorter problem-drinking histories, are less likely to perceive themselves as different from "social drinkers," and often have greater social and occupational stability (Tucker et al., 2004; Wild, 2002). These clients frequently gravitate towards reduced drinking goals, as opposed to abstinence, and may present in a state of "motivational conflict" about changing their drinking.

Brief Screening and Assessment of Problem Alcohol Use

As GSC is tailored to individuals with mild-to-moderate levels of alcohol and other drug dependence, careful screening is vital. Individuals with more severe levels of dependence generally require more intensive approaches incorporating coping-skills training and abstinence goals. Thus, using a brief measure of substance dependence can be very helpful in determining who is most suitable for GSC treatment. Examples include the SADD (Short-form Alcohol Dependence Data Questionnaire, Raistrick, Dunbar and Davidson, 1983, www.paihdelinkki.fi/english/tests/sadd_e1.htm), the

ADS (Alcohol Dependence Scale, Ross, Gavin, & Skinner, 1990, www.niaaa.nih.gov/publications/ads.htm), and the AUDIT (Saunders et al., 1993, www.niaaa.nih.gov/publications/audit.htm). In addition, a good instrument for drug-use screening is the DAST (Skinner, 1983, www.projectcork.org/clinical_tools/pdf/DAST.pdf).

One of the most straightforward screening methods is to make talking about substance use a routine practice with every person seeking help in an EAP context. This means establishing a rapport with the employee, asking questions to learn whether there are reasons to be concerned about alcohol or other drug use, acting upon those concerns, identifying and working within the employee's stage of change, and responding in suitable ways. It is helpful to begin with a question about the person's substance-use history; if alcohol or other drugs have *ever* been used, ask about current use; if the person reports current use, ask about any concern(s) caused by use in the past year. One of the best indicators of the level of alcohol-use dependence is whether an employee or family member has a history of severe alcohol withdrawal, such as hallucination, seizures, convulsions, or and/or delerium tremors 24 to 48 hours after stopping drinking. An employee who reports having had any of these symptoms would not be a suitable candidate for GSC.

Low-Risk Drinking Guidelines

In discussing an employee's use of alcohol, it is useful to share information about what low-risk drinking means. The above quantity/frequency questions can be interpreted in relation to recommended guidelines for low-risk drinking. Research-based advice on what is meant by a "standard drink," as well as suggested daily and weekly drinking limits for both women and men, can, when delivered in a neutral, non-judgmental style, help motivate an individual to examine his or her own drinking. It is recommended that women drink no more than nine standard drinks in any week, and no more than two standard drinks on any single day. Guidelines for men are a maximum of 14 standard drinks per week, and no more than three standard drinks per day (Ashley et al., 1997).

What about Employees Who Don't Want to Change?

Motivational Interviewing (MI), developed by Dr. William Miller (Miller & Rollnick, 2002), represents one way to employ a non-judgmental approach to talking about substance use. MI addresses how EAP counsellors can enhance clients' motivation for change. It has spread widely through the addiction field and beyond, likely due to its clinical utility, research support, and congruence with core values of counselling and therapy. These core values include unconditional positive regard, starting where the client is, and mutual respect (Rogers, 1951). Instead of framing people's reluctance to seek treatment as denial, Miller notes that all people are ambivalent about changing any behaviour. Confronting people who are already ambivalent simply leads to greater resistance.

Research on motivation and change has found a number of active ingredients in motivational interventions, including:

- providing personalized feedback to the employee about his or her substance-use consequences, costs, and/or risk;
- encouraging employees to take responsibility for change;
- offering neutral, non-judgmental advice;
- offering a menu of treatment alternatives;
- using empathic listening and reflection; and
- believing in the individual's ability to come up with solutions and make changes.

The GSC intervention incorporates these principles through the use of clinical assessment feedback, goal choice, and self-generated strategies for change.

In terms of counselling style, practitioners using GSC are encouraged to adopt the MI stance of emphasizing personal choice and control and working in partnership with the client. The five key principles of motivational interviewing summarize the essence of this approach (Miller and Rollnick, 2002):

i)   Avoid arguing. Emphasizing personal choice and control can be helpful in this—"Yes, it may be that you're not ready to make a change in your drinking. What you do about your drinking is entirely your choice. It's really up to you."

ii) Express empathy. Allow the employee to know that he or she has been understood—"so you're feeling angry because your supervisor made you come here and talk with me today, and you're not even convinced that you have a problem with alcohol."

iii) Develop discrepancy between the employee's or family member's behaviour and personal values—"so on the one hand you tell me that you want to be a good parent, but you also mention that you can't get up in the mornings to help your son because you're hung over. How does that fit for you?"

iv) Roll with resistance. Meet resistance with reflection: "So you're not so sure that you even need to see an EAP counsellor."

v)   Support self-efficacy. Be supportive and optimistic that the employee or family member is capable of making the change—"I have seen other people succeed before with this exact level of use."

Of course, there is a great deal more to motivational interviewing than it is possible to address here. Readers interested in learning more about the MI approach are encouraged to explore the Motivational Interviewing Website (www.motivationalinterview.org), as well as Miller's online publication *Enhancing motivation for change in substance abuse treatment* (1999, available at www.motivationalinterview.org/library/TIP35/TIP35.htm).

Guided Self-Change Treatment

Once an individual has been screened and assessed, and a determination of a low-to-moderate level of substance dependence has been made, GSC treatment can be proposed as a possible option. It is important to acknowledge that this approach is not for everyone: some employees may want or need longer-term therapy to address underlying issues, or the emphasis on written, take-home exercises may not be suitable for those with literacy issues or cognitive impairments. In addition, because GSC does not teach coping skills, but rather, relies on the internal resources of the individual, some may require a more intensive and supportive intervention. Nonetheless, for cognitively intact employees and family members of low-to-moderate dependence, the brevity and straightforwardness of this approach can make it an appealing and accessible treatment option within the confines of an EAP counselling environment, particularly those with a counselling cap.

GSC Session One: Making the Decision to Change

This session is focused on encouraging the client to consider his or her reasons for change, along with the impact that substance use has had on his or her life. Clients are asked to complete a brief reading highlighting the process in which people engage when initiating any behaviour change. GSC attempts to reduce the stigma associated with substance-abuse problems by avoiding labelling change, and by viewing ambivalence about change as normal. Indeed, the GSC program is presented as a general problem-solving approach that can helpfully be applied to other areas of a person's life in which change is being considered.

The readings and homework assignments are designed to communicate the treatment approach in an understandable and consistent way, and to provide a framework for clients to evaluate and change their behaviour. In addition, these exercises are constantly available to both client and counsellor, providing useful clinical material for discussion during the session. Compliance can indicate a person's commitment to making serious efforts to change.

In the first exercise, clients are asked to list their three major reasons for change, and then to weigh the costs and benefits of both continuing to use substances and changing their current substance use. Samples of this tool are illustrated in Figure 13.2. The objective is to elicit the client's own best arguments for change, and to build on this during the treatment session. By highlighting the costs and consequences of continued substance use, one may be able to "tip the balance" in favour of change.

Once the client has identified her reasons for change and considered the attendant costs and benefits, she is asked to set a drinking- or other drug-use goal. Clients' goal-setting is accompanied by a discussion of low-risk drinking guidelines (Figure 13.2), as well as contra-indications to reduced drinking goals. Clients who are pregnant, those currently taking prescription medication, people with certain medical conditions, such as diabetes, seizure disorder, peptic ulcer or gastritis, heart disease, or liver disease, should be advised that abstinence is necessary. In addition, clients with a legal prohibition against drinking, or those with a risk of adverse social consequences such as serious conflict with a partner, should also be advised that an abstinence goal is their best option.

Of course, many individuals for whom *any* drinking or drug use constitutes a risk may decide to reduce, as opposed to eliminate, use of a given substance. In these cases, a harm-reduction approach may be the EAP counsellor's best avenue, where a reduction in use is regarded as a step closer to the ideal goal of abstinence. The validity of this approach has been recognized for some time, with the recognition that although a uniform approach to client goal-setting may be simplest, the concept of different goals for different individuals fits best with the heterogeneity of alcohol problems (Institute of Medicine, 1990).

Goal-setting in GSC treatment asks employees and family members to determine whether abstinence or reduced drinking will fit best for them. If reduced drinking is selected as a goal, clients are asked to specify the quantity and frequency of substance use, the circumstances under which they will or will not drink or use other drugs, the importance of their goal, rated on a scale from zero to 100 percent, and their confidence in achieving their goal, also rated on a scale of zero to 100 percent. In addition, advice is given about low-risk drinking guidelines, and contra-indications to reduced drinking. Clients also have an opportunity to revisit their substance-use goal towards the end of the GSC treatment program.

Figure 13.2: Reasons for change and decisional balance

Reasons for change

Making a commitment to meeting your drinking goal is important to your success. Sometimes, it's easy to forget why you're making the change, so write down your reasons and use this as a reminder to yourself when things seem tough!

The most important reasons why I want to change my drinking or drug use are:

1. _____

2. _____

3. _____

Decision to Change
Worksheet

	Changing my current alcohol use	Continuing to use alcohol in the same way
Benefits		
Costs		

Adapted from: Centre for Addiction and Mental Health (CAMH), 1998b.

Finally, clients complete a "Drinking/Drug-Use Diary" each day, in which they record any substance use, triggers, and/or cravings. Self-monitoring forces individuals to be aware of their drinking or other drug use, and safeguards against distorted perceptions about use. This weekly record also provides client and counsellor with a picture of substance use throughout treatment, provides a basis for evaluating whether a change in substance use is occurring, and allows for a discussion of alcohol or other drug use without awkwardness. Figure 13.3 illustrates a simplified version of a "Daily Diary" that can be used in GSC treatment.

GSC Session 2: Looking at Where and When you Drink or Use Drugs
One of the benefits of the GSC approach is the way in which each session builds on the one before. In screening and assessment, clients are given personalized feedback about their alcohol- or other drug-use patterns and consequences, helping to raise individual awareness of the costs of continued substance use. The assessment stage is followed by exercises and discussion aimed at building motivation for change. This entails asking clients to articulate their reasons for changing their substance use, weighing the pros and cons of changing their use, or continuing to use alcohol or other drugs in the same way, and setting a substance-use goal. This next session is designed to help clients analyze the situations in which they are at greatest risk for problem use, and to identify past, present, and future consequences.

In the second session, an important theme is the notion of a realistic view of recovery, where the emphasis is placed on the long-term process of behaviour change. Figure 13.4 illustrates this point using the "Mount Recovery" diagram, where slips are regarded as opportunities for learning from mistakes and continuing to make progress towards one's goal. In other words, a temporary return to problem substance use is not viewed as a failure, but rather, as a small "bump in the path" towards long-term change. A brief reading orients the client to this realistic perspective, and sets the stage for a discussion about substance-use triggers and consequences.

The exercise "Looking at Where and When You Drink/Use Drugs" (Figure 13.5) asks individuals to identify the three most typical situations over the past year that were associated with their problem substance use. The first step is providing a brief description of one of the three most serious high-risk situations, and then outlining the specific triggers usually associated with this situation. Employees and family members are also asked to report the types of consequences usually associated with the risk situation, including both short- and long-term consequences, as well as the positive and negative outcomes they have experienced. The rationale for this assignment is that an analysis of trigger situations leads to a better

Figure 13.3: Daily Diary

Daily Diary

Keeping a diary is a key part of any behaviour-change program. It gives you accurate details about the behaviour you want to change, and can also help you to identify high-risk situations. This diary can also help you to see when you aren't likely to engage in this behaviour, and to identify what was different about those days. Keeping a diary takes time and commitment, but research has shown that simply keeping track of a behaviour can lead to change!

What is your goal for this week?

Date	Behaviour	Describe the situation (e.g., were you alone or with others, at home or in a social setting, etc.)	Thoughts and feelings (What were you thinking and feeling in this situation?)
Monday			
Tuesday			
Wednesday			
Thursday			
Friday			
Saturday			
Sunday			

Adapted from: Centre for Addiction and Mental Health (CAMH), 1998b.

Figure 13.4: Mount Recovery: Hill of decisions, decisions, decisions

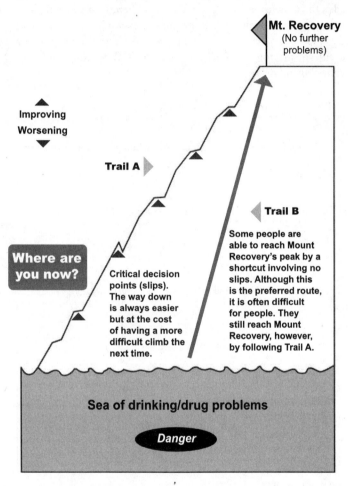

Adapted from: Centre for Addiction and Mental Health (CAMH), 1998b.

understanding of what individuals need to anticipate and plan for. Specific examples are used, as these tend to elicit richer detail than more generalized descriptions. Identifying all consequences is desirable, as this facilitates clients' recognition that while short-term consequences may be positive, the longer-term costs are almost universally negative. This exercise echoes the decisional-balance assignment discussed in GSC Session One, but adds the dimension of triggering events, thereby introducing clients to the concept of planning for risk situations. Session Three then focuses on the development of concrete strategies for avoiding or coping with triggering events in the future. Finally, as in each GSC session, the Daily Diary is reviewed and discussed.

Figure 13.5: Looking at where and when you drink/use drugs

High-risk situation: _____

1. Briefly describe one of your three most serious high-risk situations.

2. Describe as specifically as possible the types of triggers usually associated with this situation.

3. Describe as specifically as possible the types of consequences usually associated with this situation (immediate and delayed consequences, and positive and negative consequences).

How often did this type of situation occur in the past year? What percentage of your total problem substance use over the past year occurred in this type of situation? _____%

Adapted from: Centre for Addiction and Mental Health (CAMH), 1998b.

GSC Session 3: Exploring Options for Action

In Session Two clients were asked to identify the situations which presented the greatest risk for problem drinking or other drug use. Session Three asks them to come up with as many alternative behavioural options as possible, and then to develop a concrete action plan *for* each of the three risk situations they identified in the previous session. Figure 13.6 illustrates this exercise, which is in two parts. The most commonly occurring trigger situation is identified first, and then at least four alternative responses to this situation are identified. For example, many clients state that they are at risk for heavy drinking when they come home after a stressful day at work. Options in this situation might include: i) doing something constructive after work to unwind instead of coming directly home; ii) coming home right after work but not drinking heavily; iii) getting together with a supportive friend; or iv) taking steps to reduce stress during the day at work.

In assisting employees to evaluate their options, it is helpful to consider their respective outcomes. For example, not using substances and acting constructively can be expected to have a beneficial outcome, while not using substances but not acting constructively would likely lead to a harmful outcome. Similarly, using alcohol or other drugs, but not to excess, would lead to a beneficial outcome, and using alcohol or other drugs to excess would lead to a harmful outcome. In deciding on the best options, clients may find it helpful to consider their readiness to see the options through, the degree to which some might be easier to accomplish than others, and the personal costs of each option. After generating a number of options and thinking about their likely outcomes and feasibility, clients are asked to select their best option, along with a second-best option as a back-up.

Once the best and second-best options are selected, a concrete plan of action is formulated for both. In the example above, an individual might choose number two as the best option, and number one as the second-best option. That is, coming home right after work but not drinking heavily is the best option in this example, and engaging in an alternative after-work activity is seen as the second-best option. The next, and most important, step is to come up with a plan for carrying out each of these options. Thus, the steps in an action plan for the option "coming home from work but not drinking heavily" might include:

- Getting rid of alcohol in the house;
- Renting a movie or buying a good book;
- Preparing a favorite supper;
- Having a warm bath.

Figure 13.6: Exploring options for action

Options Worksheet

Describe four options and their likely consequences for your high-risk situation:

Options ("If I...")	Consequences ("Then...")
1.	
2.	
3.	
4.	

Now, select your best option and your second-best option for handling this high-risk drinking situation:

My best option is: #_____ My second-best option is: #_____

Please go on to complete the Action Plan Worksheet for this high-risk situation.

Action Plan Worksheet

High-risk situation:

For each of your best two options, describe an Action Plan to help you achieve your goal.

Best option: _____

ACTION PLAN

_____

_____

_____

_____

_____

Second-best option: _____

ACTION PLAN

_____

_____

_____

_____

_____

How often did this type of situation occur in the past year? What percentage of your total problem substance use over the past year occurred in this type of situation? _____%

Adapted from: Centre for Addiction and Mental Health (CAMH), 1998b.

Often, the greatest challenge in Session Three lies in the development of a practical, realistic, and feasible Action Plan. When additional GSC sessions are requested by an employee, it is usually because further refinement and practice of the Action Plan are needed.

During this third GSC session, it is also important to discuss the Daily Diary, and to review the employee's or family member's progress towards his or her goal. If slips occur, these can be analyzed in light of the risk situations outlined in the previous session. In addition, referring to the "Mount Recovery" metaphor can help frame these lapses as learning opportunities on the path towards long-term behaviour change.

GSC Session 4: Steps toward the Future

This final session is an opportunity to revisit a number of key elements of GSC treatment, and to assess the client's need for further support and follow-up. After Session Three, clients are asked to complete a second Goal Statement, which allows them to evaluate the feasibility and reasonableness of the goal they initially set. For example, some clients initially choose to moderate their drinking, but over the course of treatment many find that it is easier not to drink at all. Others may further reduce the consumption limits they first set for themselves as alcohol or other drug use begins to play a diminished role in their lives. By examining the first and second Goal Statements, one can gain a greater perspective on the efficacy of GSC treatment, as employee and EAP counsellor compare the client's confidence and importance ratings for the goal. Ideally, both will have increased; however diminished confidence is not uncommon, and may signal a more realistic appraisal of a client's ability to achieve her goal.

Employees or family members are also asked to revisit the Decisional Balance exercise they completed in Session One of GSC treatment. This task asked clients to anticipate the costs and benefits of changing substance-use patterns. It is now possible to look at the extent to which these costs and benefits actually "came true." Questions to ask of the employee include whether the anticipated costs were as significant as she thought, and whether there were any additional, unanticipated benefits to quitting or reducing substance use. This is also an opportunity to review the client's current motivation for change, and what else may be needed to continue to progress towards her goal.

Perhaps most important, this session presents an opportunity to re-examine the Action Plans completed in Session Three. In order to ensure sufficient time to experience and practice coping with risk situations, some clients find it helpful to schedule two to three weeks between these last two sessions. Some clients may decide that one or two additional sessions are needed in order to further refine their Action Plans. Of course, substance-use problems generally take considerable time to develop, and will not likely be completely resolved in a few brief sessions. Therefore, the end of GSC treatment should be regarded as the beginning of new approaches to substance-use triggers and risk situations.

The main goal of GSC treatment is for a client to ultimately become his own therapist, continuing to use the tools learned throughout treatment. Due to the brevity of the GSC approach, which fits the structure of some EAP contracts, it is advisable to contract for at least one or two additional telephone follow-up contacts. Setting an appointment one month and then three months post-treatment is reasonable in order to check in with the employee or the family member to assess whether continued progress is being made. It is also quite common for underlying issues to emerge during treatment. In such cases, a referral to some other specialized program can be made.

Implications for EAP Practice

The brief-treatment model outlined in this chapter is suitable for individuals with low to moderate levels of alcohol- and other drug-use severity. Careful screening and assessment are important, as people with more severe levels of dependence generally require more intensive treatment approaches. However, GSC represents a treatment option tailored for a historically underserved segment of the population. As most people with low levels of severity never cross the threshold of specialized addiction programs, the ability to work with individuals in the workplace setting in which they present is key.

The GSC approach is designed to elicit and amplify an employee's own best reasons for change. Furthermore, employees guide the treatment process by setting their own goals, identifying risk situations, and generating plans for alternative action steps. The EAP counsellor's role is more consultative than directive, giving feedback, encouraging elaboration, and providing relevant information. This can be a challenge to both clients and counsellors, who may be accustomed to a more prescriptive approach to substance-abuse treatment. However, GSC adopts a pragmatic perspective on change, acknowledging that, in the end, clients will adopt goals and strategies of their own choosing. An openness to clients' goals and priorities is also consistent with culturally competent practice principles that emphasize respect and autonomy (Straussner, 2002).

Due to its brevity and flexibility, GSC can be easily incorporated into an EAP setting. It is preferable to carry out brief screening with all clients who present to an EAP, regardless of whether or not they present with substance-use problems. This is because individuals with low to moderate levels of severity may not even be aware that their substance use poses any significant risks. Individuals who then are identified as being at risk can be offered a more intensive assessment to explore the costs and consequences of their substance use, and their interest in engaging in a brief, structured treatment.

The GSC treatment model will ideally provide EAP professionals with a set of additional tools for use with clients experiencing substance-use problems. The tools can be applied as a cohesive treatment protocol, or used piecemeal as the need arises. In addition, EAP counsellors working with diverse client populations have found it helpful to adapt the tools to best fit the unique needs of their clients. Thus, GSC can be used in conjunction with family or couples' counselling, as an adjunct to other therapeutic approaches, and in either group or individual form. In the end, the utility of the tools is best demonstrated by their application.

Endnotes

1.   Bond & Dryden, 2002; Bandura, 1977.
2.   Miller & Rollnick, 2002.
3.   Prochaska & Norcross, 1999; Prochaska, DiClemente, & Norcross, 1992.
4.   Berg & Miller, 1993.
5.   Bischof et al., 2003; Sobell, Sobell, & Agrawal, 2002; Tucker, 2001.

References

Ashley, M.J., Ferrence, R., Room, R., Bondy, S., Rehm, J., & Single, E. (1997). Moderate drinking and health. Implications of recent evidence, *Canadian Family Physician* 43, 1341–1343.

Babor, T.F. (1994). Avoiding the horrid and beastly sin of drunkenness: Does dissuasion make a difference? *Journal of Consulting and Clinical Psychology* 62, 1127–1140.

Bandura, A. (1977). Self-efficacy: Toward a unifying theory of behavioural change. *Psychological Review* 84(2), 191–215.

Berg, I.K. & Miller, S.D. (1992). *Working with the problem drinker: A solution-focused approach*. New York: W.W. Norton.

Bischof, G., Rumpf, H.-J., Hapke, U., Meyer, C., & John, U. (2003). Types of natural recovery from alcohol dependence: A cluster analytic approach. *Addiction* 98(12), 1737–1746

Bond, F.W. & Dryden, W. (2002). *Handbook of brief cognitive behavior therapy*. New York: Wiley.

Centre for Addiction and Mental Health (CAMH). (1998a). *Guided self-change for Employee Assistance Programs: Counsellor's manual*. Toronto: CAMH.

Centre for Addiction and Mental Health (CAMH). (1998b). *Guided self-change for Employee Assistance Programs: Client workbook*. Toronto: CAMH.

Dunn, C., Deroo, L., & Rivara, F.P. (2001). The use of brief interventions adapted from motivational interviewing across behavioral domains. *Addiction* 96(12), 1725–1742.

Heather, N. (2002). Effectiveness of brief interventions proved beyond reasonable doubt. *Addiction* 97(3), 293–294.

Institute of Medicine. *Broadening the base of treatment for alcohol problems*. Washington, DC: National Academy Press, 1990.

Marlatt, G.A. & Gordon, J.R. (eds.) (1995). *Relapse prevention*. New York: Guilford Press.

Martin, G.W., Herie, M.A., Turner, B.J., & Cunningham, J.A. (1998). A social marketing model for disseminating research-based treatments to addictions treatment providers. *Addiction* 93(11), 1703–1715.

Martin, G., Koski-Jannes, A., & Weber, T.R. (1998). Rethinking the role of residential treatment for individuals with substance abuse problems. *Canadian Journal of Community Mental Health* 17(1), 61–77.

Miller, W.R. & Rollnick, S. (2002). *Motivational interviewing: Preparing people to change* (2nd edn). New York: Guilford Press.

Moos, R.H. & Moos, B.S. (2003). Long term influence of duration and intensity of treatment on previously untreated individuals with alcohol use disorders. *Addiction* 98, 325–337.

Moyer, A., Finney, J.W., Swearingen, C.E., & Vergun, P. (2002). Brief intervention for alcohol problems: A meta-analytic review of controlled investigations in treatment-seeking and non-treatment-seeking populations. *Addiction* 97, 279–292.

Prochaska, J.O., DiClemente, C.C., & Norcross, J.C. (1992). In search of how people change: Applications to addictive behaviours. *American Psychologist* 47, 1102–1114.

Prochaska, J.O & Norcross, J.C. (1999). *Systems of psychotherapy: A trans-theoretical perspective*. Pacific Grove: Brooks/Cole.

Raistrick, D., Dunbar G., & Davidson, R. (1983). Development of a questionnaire to measure alcohol dependence, *British Journal of Addiction* 78, 89–95.

Rogers, C.R. (1951). *Client-centered therapy: Its current practice, implications, and theory*. Boston: Houghton Mifflin.

Ross, H.E., Gavin, D.R., & Skinner, H.A. (1990). Diagnostic validity of the MAST and the Alcohol Dependence Scale in the assessment of DSM-III alcohol disorders. *Journal of Studies on Alcohol* 51(6), 506–513.

Saunders, J.B., Aasland, O.G., Babor, T.F., de la Puente, J.R., and Grant, M. (1993). Development of the Alcohol Use Disorders Screening Test (AUDIT). WHO collaborative project on early detection of persons with harmful alcohol consumption. II. *Addiction* 88, 791–804.

Skinner, H.A. (1983). The Drug Abuse Screening Test. *Addictive Behaviors* 7(4), 363–371.

Sobell, L.C., Sobell, M.B, & Agrawal, S. (2002). Self-change and dual recoveries among individuals with alcohol and tobacco problems: Current knowledge and future directions. *Alcoholism: Clinical & Experimental Research* 26(12), 1936–1938.

Sobell, M.B. and Sobell, L.C. (1996). *Problem drinkers: Guided self-change treatment.* New York: Guilford.

Sobell, M.B. and Sobell, L.C. (1998). Guiding self-change. In W.R. Miller & N. Heather (eds.), *Treating addictive behaviours* (2nd edn). New York: Plenum Press.

Straussner, S.L. (2002). Ethnic cultures and substance abuse. *Counselor.* December, 2002, 34–38.

Tucker, J.A. (2001). Resolving problems associated with alcohol and drug misuse: Understanding relations between addictive behavior change and the use of services. *Substance Use & Misuse: Special Issue: Natural recovery research across substance use* 36(11), 1501–1518.

Tucker, J. A., Vuchinich, R. E., & Rippens, P. D. (2004). Different variables are associated with help-seeking patterns and long-term outcomes among problem drinkers. *Addictive Behaviors* 29(2), 433–439.

Wild, C. (2002). Personal drinking and sociocultural drinking norms: A representative population study. *Journal of Studies on Alcohol* 63(4), July, 469–475.

14

Intervention in the Workplace

Penny Lawson

Introduction

> Intervention: A caring process by which a group of people presents reality
> in a caring way to a colleague whose workplace performance suggests a
> problem with an addiction or with a compulsive behaviour.
>
> Bellwood Health Services

In the past, conventional wisdom suggested that anyone with an addiction issue had to reach his or her own *bottom* before being willing to admit that there was a problem, to become abstinent, and to accept help in the form of treatment (Glatt, 1954). That *bottom* for some meant that various elements of wellness—family, work, physical health, friends, self-respect, and in extreme cases, mental health—were all lost. For some the *bottom* also meant that those most closely associated with the person, especially children in the family, were also the most deeply affected. Recovery from any *bottom* is possible, but the deeper it is, the greater the shame, and the more difficulties there are to overcome. Addiction will often continue unless consequences occur that the person is unwilling to accept, and one of the mechanisms that keep addiction going is called denial or being in a state of precontemplation (Prochaska & DiClemente, 1982; 1992). This state allows the employee to minimize, intellectualize, and rationalize alcohol or other psychoactive drug use, for to think of stopping is more frightening than continuing. Some individuals with an addiction issue do not perceive reality as those around them do and they genuinely believe that they have everything under control.

Many people will change their addictive behaviour without help. Something happens such as a crisis or a meaningful experience. Many years ago a neighbour chatted with me for an hour in the driveway about his concern about his alcohol use. He decided to stop, took up golf, which then became his passion, and to the best of my knowledge he has never drunk again. Others will simply mature out of an abusive pattern of use. These people seem able to look ahead and foresee the consequences of their behaviour and make a healthy choice which enhances their overall wellness. Others, however, may need help to disengage from this destructive process.

Current practice wisdom suggests that these individuals may be assisted in having their *bottom* raised by a group of people who care about them and are willing to present to them in a caring way their concerns and observations. The advantages are many. The person abusing drugs is potentially able to progress further in recovery the sooner the misuse ends. The impact on spouses, children, families, colleagues, and the workplace is less damaging the shorter the duration of addiction. It is also accepted wisdom that it is less costly to treat and work with existing employees than it is to engage in the process of recruiting, hiring, and training new staff. Outcome studies at Bellwood Health Services demonstrated that those who worked a program in aftercare were much more likely to remain abstinent (Hambly, Wood, Levinson, & Vuksinic, 1997). Many organizations that have referred staff to a formal treatment program will also ask the center to provide reports on aftercare attendance of their employee, thereby increasing the likelihood of continued attendance. The possibility or probability of job loss acts as an incentive to begin and continue abstinence for many.

It is very difficult for most of us to express our concern for another person directly to them. When a colleague arrives in the morning smelling of alcohol or appearing impaired or hung over, few of us will comment directly to the person, or if we do it might be in the form of a joke. If we notice a pattern of absenteeism on Monday mornings, we might note it to each other, but leave dealing with it to the person's direct supervisor. Frequent visits to the washroom can be excused as illness. A change in behaviour, such as increased anger, blaming others, or expressing resentment, can be dismissed as family problems. A closed door suggests the person is working on something important. Working late is also an admirable quality and suggests hard work. Generally, as employers and colleagues, we do not like to deal with unpleasant issues or topics, which might earn us an angry or rejecting response. If we do tactfully make a comment, rather than press the point, we are inclined to accept the excuse offered and leave it at that.

We may have confused ideas of what it means to be loyal, supportive, kind, and a good colleague or friend. We also typically think that it is none of our business. Perhaps we believe that there is no recovery from an addiction. All of these thoughts may keep us silent, which unwittingly allows the problem to progress. We keep hoping the person will come to his or her senses.

Issues Intervention Addresses

There are many psychoactive substances that are addictive: alcohol, cocaine, prescription sedatives and pain medication, heroin, marijuana, and other related street drugs. There are also behaviours that may become obsessive and compulsive, such as gambling, shopping, and sex, which are extremely problematic. Most of us are familiar with the signs and symptoms of the more common substances of abuse. These include a change in appearance and behaviour, a pattern of Monday/Friday absences, an increase in the amount of absenteeism, a smell of alcohol on the breath in the morning, and difficulties with money. With cocaine addiction there might be increased visits to the washroom and requests for an advance on salary. The latter is also true of compulsive gambling. In addition to requests for advances, the compulsive gambler may begin and continue to borrow money from colleagues.

With compulsive sexual behaviour there is also a range of problematic behaviours. In the case of multiple relationships or seductive-role sex, the individual might be seen to be using excessive sexual humour, sexualizing relationships, or objectifying the opposite sex, and sexual harassment charges can result. With compulsive viewing of Internet pornography the person might actually be seen to work longer hours, arriving early and staying late, often with the door closed. Many move the computer so that someone walking by or into the room cannot see the screen. A common pattern is that at home the person waits until his or her partner is asleep and then spends many hours on the computer, becoming increasingly tired over time. The individual may begin to look haggard and unkempt, and may appear to be in a trance-like state at home and at work. Often there is an obvious change in workplace performance as projects are not completed and deadlines are not met. In most of the above scenarios there is an increasing amount of resentment expressed by colleagues who have to pick up the work left by the person under duress. Furthermore, Internet pornography is relatively inexpensive, exciting, comforting, and ultimately very isolating. It is much easier to rationalize an affair with a *cybermate* than with a real person.

It is also believed that the incidence of Internet viewing of sexual explicit material is increasingly prevalent in the workplace. In 2001, ninety-eight million unique individuals visited the top five free pornography sites on the Internet. Interestingly, 70 percent of all e-porn traffic occurs during the typical work day hours of 9:00 a.m to 5:00 p.m., with a decrease during the noon hour when many people leave their office for lunch (Delmonico & Griffin, 2002). Washton (1989) reported that 70 percent of the cocaine addicts in his outpatient program also had issues of compulsive sexual behaviour. Thus, intervention for this issue and other compulsive behaviours is important, just as it is for those who are misusing and abusing alcohol and other psychoactive drugs.

The Intervention Structure

Intervention can take many forms, and be as simple as a comment from a colleague, or as impacting as a structured intervention, which includes the supervisor, colleagues, and family members. If the workplace decides to include family, it is critical not to include children or adolescents. This is an adult problem requiring an adult solution, and children and even young adults often blame themselves if the intervention is not successful. If a structured intervention has been chosen, selecting the correct team or group is critically important. Persons to consider including are the employee's direct supervisor, along with a more senior management person, if well known to the worker, and peers with direct information and concern for the individual. All should be willing participants in the intervention. The group must exclude anyone who is unable to contain their own anger as an angry confrontation simply invites defensiveness. A defensive person will have a hard time hearing what is being said, and the intervention will not be successful. In addition, it is not recommended that an employee who is junior to the person under intervention be included in the process. If the intervention does not go well, or even if it does, this imbalance of power may produce long-term workplace and interpersonal difficulties for the intervener who is in the "one down" position. It is also wise to obtain assistance and direction in the process, preferably from a trained intervener, or at the very least, plan and rehearse what will be said at the intervention.

The intervention will have been deemed necessary as a result of the person's work performance, and indeed that is what is to be primarily spoken about in the intervention. It is not the role of the workplace to diagnose the problem, but rather to identify the behaviours about which they have concern, to state clearly the reasons for suspecting an addiction or compulsive behaviour might be involved, and to ask the employee to agree to have a formal assessment conducted by a treatment centre. If treatment becomes a necessary component for the person to maintain their job, this expectation of the employer must be stated to the person at the time of the intervention.

In the actual intervention, which takes only ten to twenty minutes, one person will have been chosen as the chairperson, and this person will introduce the reason for being there, and ask that the employee just listen until everyone has finished. Each person will have written down what they want to say, starting with a statement of positive regard and followed by the factual, non-judgmental reporting of two or three incidents, about which they have concern. After everyone has spoken the chairperson will ask that an assessment take place and will speak about the consequence of non-compliance. It is important that the mood of the intervention be even, calm, and caring. The group will have anticipated excuses ahead of time and have answers for them: for example, "I can't go to treatment now, the project is due next week." The group should expect refusal to accept what has been presented, and perhaps anger, threats, and hostility, and be prepared not to react or argue with the person. Everyone confronted with the reality of their behaviour and of their life at some point must experience anger. This is a normal response to intervention and it is one of the tasks of treatment to assist the client in working through this anger. The employee may try to bargain with the team, or suggest that they can do it on their own without help. It is important that the team considers this ahead of time and decides on what is and is not negotiable. Some teams will leave it to the person to select a treatment centre, while others will have already made a tentative assessment appointment prior to commencing the intervention. If the intervention is successful, it is important that the person not be left alone; typically the employee is in a fragile emotional state, quite shaken by what has just occurred, and will require support from those closest to them.

However if the employee refuses, the consequences of non-compliance, which must be decided upon ahead of time during an intervention-planning meeting, must be clearly stated. Many employers will give the employee a few days to a week to think about their decision and arrange a second meeting at that point to hear the decision. It is also helpful if corporations have a formal policy and procedure in place regarding time away from work.

After the Intervention

The services required are typically paid through the EAP, though in some instances the employee needs to pay for some, or even all, of a specialized treatment service. After performing an intervention in the workplace, some organizations will request, and expect, a report from the treatment center on attendance for both primary care and aftercare. Some employees may agree to seek assistance but then be unco-operative with treatment staff.

Thus, as part of the intervention process, the expectations with regard to behaviour and performance upon returning to the workplace must be clearly outlined, and a review process be set in place with clear timelines.

For those employees who enter a treatment program, many residential centers will have a day of education for the supervisors or Employee Assistance professionals, and attendance at this training is beneficial for the organization. Reintegration strategies are typically discussed and expectations for the employee clearly outlined. It is especially helpful if the returning employee has at least one person who knows what has taken place, and can be a support in the initial and long-term phases of the recovery process.

Intervention is an emotionally challenging process for everyone and is usually the method of last resort. However, where other methods have failed, the intervention process has been highly successful in returning persons with addiction issues to a happy, fulfilling, and well life.

References

Delmonico, D. and Griffin, E. (2002). In the shadows of the net: An online demonstration of the assessment and treatment of cybersex. Presentation at the *National Council on Sexual Addiction and Compulsivity, 2002 National Conference*. Nashville, Tennessee.

Glatt, M.M. (1954). Group therapy in alcoholism. *British Journal of Addiction* 54(2), 133–150.

Hambly, J., Wood, S., Levinson, T., & Vuksinic, A. (1997). *A five-year examination of program outcomes, 1991–1996*. Toronto: Bellwood Health Centre.

Prochaska, J. & DiClimente, C. (1982). Stages and process of self-change in smoking: Towards an integrative model of change. *Psychotherapy* 20, 161–173.

Prochaska, J., DiClimente, C., & Norcross, J. (1992). In search of how people change: Applications to addictive behaviors. *American Psychologist* 47(9), 1102–1114.

Washton, A. (1989). Cocaine may trigger sexual compulsivity. *Journal of Drug & Alcohol Dependency* 13(6), 8.

15

Depression in the Workplace

Louise Hartley

Introduction

The economy of the early twenty-first century can be characterized as knowledge-based, with an emphasis on thought content rather than physical labour. However, at a time when mental resiliency is needed at its most, it is being severely challenged by escalating rates of job strain, burn-out, and depression. Workplaces have been changing over the past 15 years in ways that have negatively impacted employee well-being.

"Downsizing," "rightsizing," and "re-engineering" have been some of the terms used for management processes which ultimately have resulted in workers doing more with fewer resources. Most workplaces have experienced technological changes that have led to employees feeling there is "information overload," when they think about the changes wrought by e-mail, cell phones, computer linkages between home and work, and the ever-present written correspondence. A less subtle source of stress is the customer who has become more demanding. The Sears retail chain found that even when customers rated their shopping experience a nine out of ten in terms of overall satisfaction, only 33 percent were then willing to state that they would definitely recommend Sears to prospective customers. In order for that percentage rating to increase to 82 percent, the client needed to be totally satisfied (10 out of 10) with their shopping experience (Kirn, 2000).

In a 2001 study of over 30,000 Canadian employees who worked in public, private, and non-profit organizations, it was found that 58 percent reported feeling role-overload, and having inadequate time available to meet the demands in their job and their personal life; this compares with 35 percent in 1991. Increases in overall stress rose from 43 percent to 58 percent, while reported depression of mood more than doubled from 15 percent to 33 percent between 1991 and 2001 (Duxbury & Higgins, 2003).

The Development of Depression

While a certain amount of stress is required for optimal performance, the experience of workers is that when there is no break from increasing demands, prolonged duration of stress is becoming a significant health problem. It is the beginning point of a downward spiral that is experienced as increasing feelings of fatigue, difficulty concentrating and making decisions, and withdrawal from regular social activities and support. The grouping of these symptoms has become known as "burn-out." The symptomatology, however, is very close to that defined by the DSM-IV for a major depressive episode (Table 15.1). Given the stigma and oppression that are attached to any form of mental illness (Kimberley & Osmond, 2003), it is possible that the term "burn-out" was coined to give an acceptable workplace label to a condition very similar to a major depression. Figure 15.1 illustrates the relationship over time of high stress on performance.

While external factors play a critical role in the onset of job strain, burn-out, and depressed mood, a major depression is a brain disorder influenced by a combination of genetic, environmental, and neurobiological factors.

Table 15.1: Burn-out and depression symptomatology

Burn-out	Depression (DSM-IV)
Feeling empty or trapped	At least one of the following for a two-week period: depressed mood and/or loss of pleasure or interest in life activities
Depressed mood	
Low frustration tolerance	
	Plus some of the following for a total of 5 symptoms:
Inability to concentrate, make decisions	
Physical complaints (headache, muscle pain)	significant weight loss or gain, insomnia or hypersomnia nearly every day, fatigue or loss of energy nearly every day,
Interpersonal problems/withdrawal from family and co-workers	diminished ability to think, psychomotor agitation or retardation nearly every day, feelings of worthlessness or inappropriate guilt, recurrent thoughts of death

Figure 15.1: Prolonged-duration stress

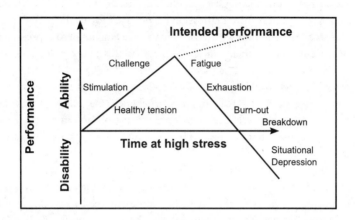

The role that each factor plays is still not clear, although depression does run in families. Children of depressed mothers have a three-fold risk for depression. While pharmacologic treatment is effective with this condition, research has still not identified that depression is the result of a reduced level of any single neurotransmitter that we can now measure.

Epidemiological Issues

Depression strikes people in their prime, typically between the ages of 24 and 44. The average age of onset is 26 years of age, which is ten years younger than a generation ago. Lifetime prevalence rates are cited as between 10 to 25 percent for women, and 5 to 12 percent for men. Depression rates in children are about equal until adolescence, when girls become twice as likely as boys to become depressed. Twenty years ago, 1.5 percent of the population experienced a depressive disorder, while it is expected that as many as 8 to 10 percent of North Americans now living will experience a major depressive episode. The World Health Organization (2001) reported that in 1996, depression was the fourth-ranked cause of disability and premature death in countries with established market economies. It is predicted that by 2020 it will be the second leading cause of disability. Two questions emerge from this epidemiological data: "Why are there gender differences?" and "Why does depression appear to be increasing?"

In attempting to understand the gender differences three possible explanations have been suggested: socialization, different manifestations for men and women, and physiology. Socialization research would suggest that males of the baby-boom generation were socialized to act out their feelings or ignore them. Given that it is estimated that half to two thirds of people who suffer from depression do not seek formal help, then perhaps males of the baby-boom generation who were taught not to express sadness because it was not manly make up most of this non help-seeking group. Therefore, the current gender differentiation is skewed by this sampling error. As socialization practices have changed over the last 50 years, and parents accepted that "real boys do cry," changes may emerge in prevalence rates. Indeed in a recent study of American College campuses, the same rate of depression was reported between male and female college students (Solomon, 2001).

It has also been postulated that men simply demonstrate depression in different ways. The typical problems that bring men to counselling centres are issues of intimacy, the compulsive need to work, or abusive behaviour. It has been contended that the core issue for each of these problems is feelings of depression that men mask: covert depression (Real, 1997). Another possible explanation for the gender difference relates to physiology. Research has shown that men synthesize serotonin about 50 percent more rapidly than women. Serotonin is one of the drugs that has been effectively use to treat depression. Thus, it has been hypothesized that men may have a natural resiliency to protect against the onset of depression (Margolis & Swartz, 1998).

The Biology of Depression

An examination of the relationship of stress and depression is relevant when considering the evidence that rates of depression are increasing. The pathology of depression shows with clarity that mind and body are not separate. Studies have found that the brains of individuals who have committed suicide have elevated levels of cortisol, and that these individuals also have enlarged adrenal glands (Solomon, 2001). It appears that individuals who have committed suicide had adrenal glands that were in "overdrive" in terms of cortisol production. It is known that stress elevates cortisol, and that as cortisol levels go up, the level of serotonin goes down. While there is no suggestion that the stress that produces cortisol causes depression, it may exacerbate a minor condition or innate predisposition and create an actual syndrome. There has also been interesting research carried out on treatment-resistant depressed patients with ketoconzaole, a cortisol-reducing medication. This medication has had a positive impact on reducing depression in 70 percent of the cases (Wolkowitz, Reus, Chan,

Manfredi, Raum, Johnson, & Canick 1999). Unfortunately ketoconzaole causes too many side effects to be attractive as a first line of treatment.

Studies have also found a relationship between depression and physical health. Once you have had a heart attack, your risk of dying from cardiovascular disease is four to six times greater if you also suffer from depression. Depression is an independent risk factor for heart disease in a range similar to that of cholesterol. Similar relationships have emerged with epilepsy, osteoporosis, and diabetes. People with these illnesses run a higher risk of disability or premature death when they are clinically depressed.

Depression can be a lethal illness. There is a 15 percent mortality rate, and one in six severely depressed people commit suicide. While women report twice as much depression, men are four times as likely to commit suicide. Robert Post of the National Institute of Mental Health reported that "while people worry about side effects from staying on medication for a lifetime, the side effects of doing that appear to be very insubstantial compared to the lethality of under treated depression" (Solomon, 2001: 80).

Recent research also indicates that for many people, depression is a life-long illness. A 15-year prospective longitudinal study of depression found that only a fifth of the sample recovered and remained continuously well, while three out of five people recovered but had further episodes; the remaining 20 percent committed suicide or were otherwise perpetually incapacitated (Andrews, 2000). Of the 60 percent who had further episodes, half relapsed within a year, and most relapsed within two years. Depressive symptoms have also been found to be present 60 percent of the time, during long-term follow-up (Judd, Mijch, Cockram, Komiti, Hoy, & Bell, 2000). One study has shown that the first episode of depression is closely linked to life events, with the second somewhat less so; by the fourth and fifth episodes, life events seem to play no part at all (Solomon, 2001). Interestingly, these major life events do not need to be negative in nature, such as loss of loved one. Major positive changes, such as a promotion or marriage, can also be a triggering event for depression.

Treating Depression

The research on the recurrence of depression has led many to suggest that depression should be managed as a chronic disease, like diabetes. In other words, if you have chosen a pharmacological intervention, you take medication for a lifetime with regular visits to your family physician to adjust the levels in order to ensure maximum functioning. If the treatment regimen is counselling, then after the initial phase of treatment you move to a dental model of treatment in which you have regular check-up visits with your counsellor—to ensure the strategies you have developed are being maintained.

While two out of three persons with depression do not seek treatment, 80 percent of people with depression can be treated effectively with medication, counselling, or a combination of the two strategies. The World Health Report (2001) compared the effectiveness of three treatment conditions (placebo, tricyclics medication, and psychotherapy) on remission of depression symptoms after three to eight months. The report states that 27 percent of the placebo sample had remission of symptoms, compared to 48 to 52 percent in the tricyclics treatment group, and 48 to 60 percent for the psychotherapy treatment group. Researchers in this area have noted that "it is striking that patients who recover from depression by means of psychotherapy show some of the same biological changes (e.g., EEG) as those who receive medication" (Solomon, 2001: 101). Indeed, for mild to moderate depression, 20 years of research have found that cognitive/ behavioural or interpersonal therapy is as effective as drugs (World Health Report, 2001). There is also some research that supports the theory that drug treatment is most effective for taking people out of depression and psychotherapy is important to prevent re-occurrence.

Unfortunately, substandard treatment for this condition remains prevalent in Canada and in the United States. The Canadian Network for Mood and Anxiety Treatment (2003) reports that antidepressant dosages persistently below the standard guideline level care are still consistently given out by family physicians. Another problem is that patients do not stay on the medication for an adequate length of time. While 80 percent of individuals respond to medication, only 50 percent respond to their first medication, and less than 25 percent of patients continue treatment for six months, which is not necessarily surprising, given the function of the medication and also some of the undesirable side effects. A large proportion stop because of the side effects related to sleep problems and sexual functioning. If medication is tried and has some impact, often patients do not return regularly enough to the treating physician to obtain further dosage adjustment, and thus only minimal or partial response is achieved. When individuals choose counselling, many clinicians fail to administer the proven standardized therapies, cognitive/behavioural, or interpersonal.

Workplace Initiatives

Apart from the human suffering that occurs with depression, the associated financial costs have a significant impact on the economy. The Global Business and Economic Roundtable on Addiction and Mental Illness (2004) estimated that mental ill health costs the Canadian economy approximately $33 billion a year. The International Labour Organization (2000) estimates that approximately 27 percent of the costs is in lost work days, while 28 percent of the costs is in decreased productivity, often called presenteeism, which results from fatigue, loss of concentration and impaired decision making. Nervous or mental conditions represent 20 to 30 percent of contemporary disability claims, with depression representing the longest average length of disability compared to other chronic medical conditions. Workplaces need to pay attention to this illness, not just because it is the "right thing to do," but also to mitigate the impact on the financial bottom line.[1]

To counteract the negative impact of increased demands and job strain, astute executive leadership is developing strategic objectives that integrate wellness initiatives into the workplace and into the business planning process. These practices create a workplace culture that fosters relationships characterized by fairness and trust. The United Kingdom has legislated a six-point stress code: this ensures that employers protect their staff from the known risks attached to such factors as high-demand and low-control jobs. While these types of preventative activities will decrease the downward spiral for many workers from job strain to burn-out or depressed mood, the illness of depression requires companies to review their identification and return-to-work processes.

Early identification of depression with referral to appropriate treatment resources is critical in mitigating the impact of this illness for the sufferer and their workplace. Employee Assistance Programs can play a central role in facilitating both aspects. Every year a plan should be developed about communication strategies for increasing employee awareness of this illness, as well as debunking certain myths about this illness, for example, that it is a personality weakness. Information should also be available to help employees and members of their families become more informed consumers, so that if they or a family member is suffering from the condition, they know the questions that should be asked to ensure that appropriate treatment regimens are being used by their family physician or counsellor.

Company personnel also need to review their return-to-work protocols. One of the biases that managers need to overcome is that mentally restored employees are second rate. The International Labour Organization (2000) found that employers who have hired mentally restored individuals report that they are higher than average in attendance and punctuality, and as good or better than other employees in motivation, quality of work, and job tenure. Another barrier that is frequently encountered in attempting to return employees who have suffered from depression is the belief that "the employee is of no use to me if they only work part-time. I want them 100 percent or not at all." Apart from the fact that employers have a duty to accommodate individuals who suffer from depression, research has indicated that complete symptom remission is not necessary to reduce serious impairment (Mintz , Mintz, & Arruda, 1992). It has also been found that there is no significant time delay between clinical improvement and increased work productivity (Simon, VonKorff, Rutter, & Wagner, 2000).

Effective return-to-work protocols ensure that timely information about the financial implications of a disability leave is given to the employee. Support in filling out the necessary paperwork in a timely manner can greatly help the depressed employee feel truly supported by their employer and the workplace. The manager needs to ensure that either they or someone from the team stays in touch with the depressed employee. This is to ensure that the employee knows the team is interested in the employee's well-being and to keep the employee up to date on changes in the department or the social "gossip," the vital social component of wellness. Keeping this link makes re-entry into the workforce much easier and more likely. Research has shown that the likelihood of returning to work decreases as time away from work increases. There is an 80 percent return rate if the absence is less than 3 months, 50 percent if less than half a year, and there is only a 20 percent return rate after one year of absence (MacDonald, 2003).

Conclusion

In summary, the changes that have occurred in the workplace over the past 15 years have led to a marked increase in the number of employees who are experiencing a range of behavioural health problems and impaired wellness. While job strain, depressed mood, and burn-out can be viewed as falling on a continuum of increasingly serious symptomatology, depression is a distinct illness whose etiology is multi-determined. However, all four conditions have an impact on a company's financial bottom line, both through the direct costs of absenteeism and drug-plan benefits, and the harder-to-measure costs associated with presenteeism. Workplaces need to examine their values and operating practices to ensure that they are developing a culture that promotes employee's wellness. They also need to ensure that they are informing their employees and employees' families about depression as part of routine EAP practice. This communication must include information about both symptoms and effective treatments. It must debunk myths that depression is a condition about which an individual should be ashamed, or that it is a personality weakness. Finally, company personnel need to review their return-to-work policy and procedures in order to ensure that employees return to work in a manner that promotes their wellness and allows them to positively contribute at work, at home, and in the community.

Endnote

1. See also Chapter 3 on Disability Management.

References

Andrews, G. (2000). Should depression be managed as a chronic disease? www.depressionet.com.au/research/rsch_chronic.html.

Canadian Network for Mood and Anxiety Treatment. (2003). *Depressed? Anxious?* www.canmat.org/depress/three/depresstop.htm.

Duxbury, L. & Higgins, C. (2001). *Work–life balance in the new millenium: Where are we? Where do we need to go? Discussion Paper No. W/12*. Ottawa: Canadian Policy Research Network,

Global Business and Economic Roundtable on Addiction and Mental Health. (2004). *Top business leaders endorse new mental health guidelines.* www.mentalhealthroundtable.ca.

International Labour Organization. (2000). *Mental health in the workplace.* Geneva: International Labour Organization.

Judd, F.K., Mijch, A., Cockram, A., Komiti, A., Hoy, J., & Bell, R. (2000). Depressive symptoms reduced in individuals treated with HAART: A longitudinal study. *Australian & New Zealand Journal of Psychiatry* 34(6), 1015–1021 .

Kimberly, M. D. & Osmond, M.L. (2003). Concurrent disorders and social work interventions. In R. Csiernik and W.S. Rowe (eds.), *Responding to the oppression of addiction: Canadian social work perspectives.* Toronto: Canadian Scholars' Press.

Kirn, S. (2000). *Sears Roebuck: Customer satisfaction.* Chicago: IQPC HR Measurements Conference.

Lemonic, M. (2003). The power of mood. *Time,* January 20, 37–41.

MacDonald, C. *Making an impact—Is it worth the investment?* Paper presented at The Second Annual Workplace Mental Health Summit, Toronto, 2003.

Margolis, S. & Swartz K. (1998). Sex difference in brain serotonin production. *The Johns Hopkins White Papers* #14.

Mintz, J., Mintz, L.I., & Arruda, M.J. (1992). Treatments of depression and the functional capacity to work. *Archives of General Psychiatry* 49, 761–768.

Real, T. (1997). *I don't want to talk about it—Overcoming the secret legacy of male depression.* New York: Simon & Schuster.

Simon, G., VonKorff, M., Rutter, C., & Wagner, E. (2000). A randomized trial of monitoring, feedback, and management of care by telephone to improve depression treatment in primary care. *British Medical Journal* 320, 550–554.

Solomon, A. (2001). *The noonday demon: An atlas of depression.* New York: Touchstone.

Wolkowitz, O.M., Reus, V., Chan, T., Manfredi, F., Raum, W., Johnson, R., & Canick, J. (1999). Antiglucocorticoid treatment of depression: Double-blind ketoconazole. *Biological Psychiatry* 45 (8), 1070–1074.

World Health Organization (2001). *WHO Report 2001: Mental health—New understanding, new hope.* www.who.int/whr2001/2001.

16

Grief in the Workplace:
A Practitioner's Perspective

Hilda Sabadash

Introduction

Grief is a very personal feeling, and individuals carry it differently on their way to work, during work, and returning from work. For example, when a colleague dies, some co-workers dread going to work because the connections to sadness are reinforced by the absence of the co-worker. Others want to be at work among supportive colleagues who are also grieving for the same person. Similarly, if a family member dies, going to work may be viewed as a reprieve by some family members simply because the workplace has fewer reminders of their grief. Others in a similar situation may be unable to function at work because their workplace is not perceived to be a supportive environment. This chapter discusses the range of normal grieving in the workplace and suggests supportive approaches for addressing it.

Healthy Grief

Grief is the normal and natural emotional reaction to a change or end in any familiar pattern of behaviour (James & Friedman, 2003). Although health is defined as a state of complete physical, mental, and social well-being, and not merely the absence of disease or infirmity (World Health Organization, 1946), the notion of grief is not explicit or normalized in most descriptions of health and wellness. Instead, it is hidden under labels that suggest diagnosis, treatment, and absence from work highlighted by stress, burn-out, exhaustion, or depression. However, grief is not a sickness. People who are grieving are frequently able to work if they have the necessary mutual respect and support in their workplaces.

The notions of health and wellness are visible everywhere in our society. They are supported in well-funded government programs, are featured on television, on radio, and in film and print media. Schools have a wide range of programs encouraging students to be physically active and eat healthy foods. Fundraising events are frequently based on physical activity, on walking or running for a cure or for research.

Grief, on the other hand, is largely invisible. Grieving is personal and considered to be a private process, and therefore tends not to be promoted in the same way as health and wellness. Crying is seen to be "embarrassing" and a sign of emotional weakness, rather than a natural expression of feelings of loss. Feelings that are not discussed may return at a later date (Doka 1989).

Two researchers who have contributed significantly to understanding the process of grief are Dr. Elizabeth Kübler-Ross and Dr. Theresa Rando. Kübler-Ross's (1969) five stages of grief are well known: denial, anger, bargaining, depression, and acceptance. Rando's (1993) approach, on the other hand, identifies three main phases: avoidance, confrontation, and accommodation. Other words which are sometimes used for Rando's term "avoidance" phase are shock, disbelief, "feeling numb," "being in a daze," or feeling "startled."

Most people seek help in the second phase—confrontation. At this point the shock has worn off, as several months have usually passed since the death occurred. In addition, support from community and co-workers is usually on the wane. During this phase there is also an expectation on the part of the grieving individuals and others around them that they should begin to feel stronger and "get on with their lives." However, many who are grieving are surprised to feel that their emotions can be much stronger during this second phase of confrontation than immediately after the funeral. They find that crying comes quickly and without warning: one minute they feel fairly comfortable, while the next minute, they burst into tears, and then a few minutes later they feel composed again. This quick change in feelings is not necessarily tied to stressful times: it can occur when doing daily household routines such as buying groceries or doing laundry or simply sitting at one's desk at work. A frequent phrase heard by counsellors is "I think I'm going crazy." Although understanding the stages of grief helps to ground EAP practitioners, clients are rarely interested in knowing about their particular stage of grieving. Rather, individuals typically want to hear that they are normal, that their feelings are also experienced by others who are grieving, and that they are not "going crazy" just because they feel out of control. The final stage in Rando's process, accommodation, is about re-establishment. At this phase, people are more able to go to work with confidence in their emotional state. They feel fewer emotional waves, and are able to make grounded decisions and healthy choices about how they want to shape their future working and personal lives. They generally begin to feel more in control of their lives.

Supportive Employee Assistance Programs

There is evidence that the workplace is significantly affected by grief, with 90 percent of participants in a national American study reporting that their ability to concentrate was reduced (James & Friedman, 2003). Lower productivity, including absenteeism from work and poor decision-making when at work, along with memory loss, confusion, moodiness, anxiety, and sudden fatigue during work-time were common symptoms reported by employees affected by grief. EAP staff can support grieving employees and co-workers by respecting the changes that are initiated by grieving, and offering understanding and an empathic response. Following are nine guiding principles for EAP staff, which can be used to support healthy grieving in the workplace.

i)   Normalize feelings
     Most of the grieving expressed in the workplace will be well within the normal range of bereavement. Employment Assistance Program staff need to reinforce the normalcy of grieving. Emotional responses are usually accompanied by negative connotations, and people degrade themselves for having intense feelings. Statements such as "I feel so stupid crying in front of you" are commonplace. Repetition of grounding statements and repeating words, such as "grieving, normal, healthy process, comes in waves," can assure staff that their feelings are normal and accepted.

ii) Offer emotional support
     EAP staff can clarify employees' instrumental options and needs for support, including extended time for compassionate leave, counselling for underlying issues revealed through the death and ongoing bereavement support groups. Emotional support can be provided by encouraging social interactions as simple as sharing mealtimes and breaks with co-workers. The EAP counsellor or peer-referral agent needs to keep in mind that responses to questions about how an employee is feeling can vary, depending on when the question is asked and who is doing the asking. Counsellors and referral agents need to be sensitive about which individuals should engage employees in discussions about their grief, and when is an opportune time for doing so.

iii) Recognize variability in performance
      During a typical day, a colleague can be very efficient in the morning
      and lose the ability to concentrate in the afternoon. Emotions
      can surface quickly with no apparent cause. By late afternoon,
      the employee may be able to resume a task and meet an expected
      deadline. Some days, sleeplessness and lack of appetite may affect
      the performance of a grieving worker. Grieving comes in waves and
      dissipates with no regular pattern, often leaving an individual drained
      and frustrated. Individuals who have experienced the death of a
      family member frequently report that six months after the event, the
      intensity of their emotions is similar to what they felt the day of the
      funeral. If work involves stressful calculations or decisions, it may
      be wise for EAP staff to offer an unobtrusive quality-control check
      for a period of time.

iv)   Address safety concerns
      Driving is a significant safety issue, as people who are grieving may
      be overwhelmed by their emotions and unable to focus on the task at
      hand. Crying while driving is common, as people often unexpectedly
      develop intense feelings when moving from their workplace to their
      home or vice versa. In addition, many people feel that their cars
      are safe places to experience, and work through, strong emotions.
      EAP staff can offer to set up car pools or encourage people to
      travel together to and from work using public transportation when
      possible.

v)   Explore opportunities for spiritual support
      Spiritual support is not always religious or based on a specific faith.
      Questions such as "Why me, God?" need to be expressed and do
      not always require an answer. Sometimes commenting that many
      people ask similar questions can confirm the normalcy of the
      reflection. Knowing clergy who offer spiritual support to those who
      are hurting may be beneficial at this time. Office workers may prefer
      not to attend funeral ceremonies of co-workers of different faiths
      and also may not verbalize the true reason for their absence. Respect
      for differences is required in these situations.[1]

vi)   Avoid a teaching/preaching mode
      It can be humbling for EAP staff, both professional and peer, to
      accept the fact that no one can take the pain away from the person
      expressing sorrow. The emotions of a grieving individual in many
      ways represent the connection between the co-worker and the person
      who died, and need to be respected. This respect is demonstrated

by the support a counsellor or peer-referral agent may offer. Often, a silent and supportive presence may be enough. Avoid sentences that begin with "you should," "you should not," "why don't you," as these may be perceived as strong verbal suggestions or even threats. Beginning sentences with the word "I" or "others have felt comfort with" gives the listener a choice as to whether suggested ideas may be comforting or not.

vii) Communicate with colleagues about the need for mutual support
Respectful reflection about the person who has died is a healthy thing to do with co-workers. Naming the person who died is also beneficial, although some people may shy away from this and use pronouns such as "he" or "she" instead of the actual name. Reminiscing does not have to be a sad time. Off-site eulogies can be a healthy way to share grief time. Co-workers can frequently recall funny circumstances when unable to concentrate, and re-telling memorable tales is common. Golf games "in memory of" offer a supportive environment to share feelings. "S/he used to, I remember when, that irritating habit," are common testimonials when memories surface. All these things offer permissible check-ins for co-workers to support one another, particularly if it was a sudden, tragic, or workplace-based death. Some offices have a wall of plaques or a memory book that is seen as a shrine of some kind to the person who died. Co-workers need permission to do what offers comfort. This may be as individual as "her special pen" in a co-worker's desk, or a group activity such as planting a tree or donating to a charity on a one-time or ongoing basis.

viii) Recognize the potential for substance abuse
Increased smoking, alcohol or other drug intake, both licit and illicit, are all common methods used to dull the pain of bereavement. If these methods are brought into the workplace, managers need to be very clear about policies for maintaining safety and the policies regarding informal or formal use of the EAP. Changes in stress levels, such as moving a worker temporarily away from public interactions to elsewhere in the workplace, may lessen the need for reliance upon a psychoactive substance. It helps to be aware of changes in workers' daily living patterns, such as adjusted levels of medication to control anxiety attacks or enhance sleeping. Such changes may explain different levels of alertness and responsiveness during long meetings, and it can be useful for EAP staff to relate this information to supervisors and colleagues in a general way.

ix) Pay attention to language
     The following phrases, although commonly used, just don't work
     well with people who are grieving. A general rule is to avoid direct
     advice, philosophical statements, or popular maxims. Many of these
     phrases are used on television or in films in scenes where grief is
     exploited to spike an emotional response—they're not appropriate
     in real life.

          I know how you feel
          Get over it
          S/he has no pain now
          S/he is in a better place, with the angels now
          This is God's will
          You have other children to live for
          You should take a trip and get away
          Boys don't cry
          You look so strong
          You are the man/woman of the family now (after a parent has
            died).
          At least it was quick
          That's all s/he would have wanted
          You look like your mom/dad (while standing at the casket).

Benefits of Grieving

While grieving can be a very sad time, it can also have positive effects.
Funerals, memorial services, and informal gatherings enable those attending
to reflect on the positive and nurturing aspects of a deceased person's life,
and this frequently ends up being a very comforting experience for all.
In addition, these gatherings can also provide opportunities for personal
insights about life for those who are there to be supportive of immediate
family and friends, such as, "It really made me think about what's important
to me and how I am choosing to spend my time."

EAP staff are in the fortunate position of being able to offer thoughtful
and sensitive support to grieving staff. This support involves normalizing
reactions and feelings and observing enhanced self-efficacy as individuals
in the workplace come to terms with their grief and take control of their
futures. Healthy grieving is an innate and essential part of personal wellness
both in the workplace and the fullness of everyday life.

Endnote

1. The role and significance of spirituality in the workplace is explored further in Chapter 25.

References

Doka, K. (1989). *Disenfranchised grief, recognizing hidden sorrow.* Toronto: Lexington Books.

James, J. W. & Friedman, W. (2003). *The grief index: The hidden annual costs of grief in America's workplace.* Sherman Oaks, California: The Grief Recovery Institute Educational Foundation, Inc.

Kübler-Ross, E. (1969). *On death and dying.* New York: Macmillan.

Rando. T. (1993). *Treatment of complicated mourning.* Champaign, Illinois: Research Press.

World Health Organization. (1946). *Constitution.* New York.

17

The Impact of EAP-Based Mediation Services on Employees, Families, and the Workplace

David W. Adams

Introduction

The opening chapter of this volume considers how today's employees, at home and at work, are prone to the intrusion of systemic stressors that have an impact on their ability to maintain their health, wellness, and competence in coping with the challenges of daily living. In order to be effective, efficient, and competitive, EAPs, as providers of services to employees, their families, and their employers, have been required to broaden their focus and expand their mandate. They have been encouraged to be in tune with societal needs and expectations generated by lifestyles, community influences, and the workplace, replete with its diverse cultures, values, mandates, and *modus operandi*. Within the plethora of North American EAP service-delivery models, actively and astutely applied mediation skills are an integral component of client services. Mediation practices may be an inclusive and unobtrusive component of everyday counselling, or marketed as specialized fee-for-service initiative. This chapter explores the process of mediation: the mediator's role, training, values, and skills; the concepts of open and closed mediation; and three specific types of mediation relevant to EAPs. These include informal (everyday) mediation, formal (fee-for-service) family mediation, and formal (fee-for-service employer-funded) Alternative Dispute Resolution (ADR).

The Process of Mediation and the Mediator's Role

Broadly defined, mediation is a process in which disputing or disagreeing parties engage a mutually acceptable impartial third party to help them obtain an agreement to resolve or reconcile their differences (Landau, Bartoletti, & Mesbur, 1997). Fundamental to mediation is the recognition that the parties involved are responsible for making and owning all decisions reached. As a facilitator, process guide, monitor, and recorder of mutually agreed-upon decisions, the mediator helps to move parties through the process at their own pace. Enabling the process to evolve gradually so that each party has an equal opportunity to participate, buy into, and be satisfied with the outcome is essential for both the acceptance of the agreement and maintenance of its terms in the future. In order to be effective, the mediator must ensure prior to beginning the process that the parties participating have both the ability to mediate, and a clear, unfettered mandate to make lasting decisions. They must also be free from the potential interference by external forces that can negate a successful outcome. The mediator must also be able to keep the participants on track, ensure that they all have the opportunity to understand and explore in depth mutually identified problem-solving alternatives, and make certain that all parties genuinely anticipate that a resolution or reconciliation of differences will be the end result.[1]

The Mediator's Training, Values, and Skills

Mediation skills are not owned by a specific discipline, but are integrated into the diverse clinical skills of an applied profession such as social work, law, or psychology (Timms & Timms, 1977; Adams, 1982; Thompson, 2000). They may also be a component of labour studies, or informal on-the-job training of company or union personnel, or the formal or informal training of business negotiators. Recently, mediation has also become a diploma or degree program in undergraduate studies at some Canadian post-secondary institutions, where the major focus is on learning and completion of a practicum that requires learners to apply mediations skills in real-life situations. Such training is also available through post-professional continuing-education programs operated by both public and private institutions and businesses. This diversity of academic learning and skill-development opportunities is reflective of the popularity of this gentle, non-coercive, self-directed approach to problem-solving as an alternative to litigated or arbitrated settlements. It has become an acceptable approach to the settlement of both family, business, and potentially litigation-related disputes. In brief, regardless of the mediation forum, the mediator must be able to be:

i)   neutral and remain so during the entire process;
ii) non-judgmental;
iii) able to fully understand the system in which the dispute arises;

iv) willing to clarify the details of the dispute and rationale for mediation prior to beginning the process;

v) convinced that all parties are free of coercion or coercive intent and able to make and implement the decisions contained in the agreement reached;

vi) in charge of selecting a neutral site for the mediation deliberations to take place;

vii) prepared to establish the ground rules, boundaries, structural frameworks, and methodologies clearly, and ensure that these are communicated to all parties prior to initiating any part of the process. A written contract signed by all parties is also essential in ensuring that everyone participating is on side. The contract is often signed during a pre-mediation educational session;

viii) satisfied that a reconciliation or resolution of the differences cited by the parties in their initial delineation of the request to mediate can be achieved and sustained;

ix) knowledgeable about the intent of the parties regarding how any written documentation may be used; and,

x) clear about the mediator's own expectations concerning the use and dissemination of any documentation the mediator creates at any point in the process.

Is the Mediation Open or Closed?

In providing mediation services in two of the three types of mediation discussed, the mediator must establish whether the mediation is open or closed. If open, some or all of the details of both informal and formally designated mediations may be used in other legal forums. If some or all of the issues in any mediation are not resolved or those that have allegedly been resolved are legally disputed at a later date, the mediator can be required by the lawyers representing any of the participants, or a judge or other form of arbitrator, to participate in future legal proceedings. The mediator could be required to describe transactions within the mediation process in detail and defend his or her actions (Landau, Bartoletti, & Mesbur 1997). For this author, closed mediation expectations, clearly documented in a contract signed by all parties, are a much more desirable choice. In closed mediations, all details of the entire mediation process including the actions of the mediator and everyone participating remain private and may not be used in any other setting. Only the details contained within the mediator's unsigned final written report or *Memorandum of Understanding* are available to third parties. This memorandum contains outcome information regarding issues resolved or reconciled and, when appropriate, may briefly mention issues in which resolution or reconciliation was not achieved.

Three Type of Mediation

Informal mediation as a component of EAP counselling services.
In some situations the EAP counsellor has an opportunity to informally mediate and enable two or more clients to resolve or reconcile a specific mutually defined problem. This type of mediation requires the willingness of each client to set aside power differences, make mutually agreeable decisions based on needs and interests, and agree that these decisions will be respected and govern future conduct. The mediator may or may not be willing or required to establish a written contract or document the decisions and conditions of the resolution or reconciliation. Participation in this type of mediation is always voluntary and, depending on the mediator's needs, may be open or closed. In some instances, for liability reasons, EAPs as the counsellor's employer may insist on a written contract. If the mediation is a component of regular contracted EAP services of six or more counselling hours, and is skillfully administered, the entire involvement should not be expected to require more service delivery hours than the average time consumed by a series of problem-solving contacts with non-mediating clients. The following case offers one brief illustrative example of an informal mediation.

Case Example: Paula, Andy, and Margaret—Siblings in Conflict
Paula, Andy, and Margaret are all adult children of seventy-nine-year-old Louise, who is in the final stages of terminal cancer. Two years ago when she was diagnosed, Louise was worried that if she gave Paula, her most responsible and practical child, her Powers of Attorney, her other two children would be upset. Consequently, she persevered so that her lawyer constructed the legal documents to grant equal personal care and financial Powers of Attorney to each of her children. Unfortunately, as Louise's condition began to deteriorate, her previous decision created unforeseen distress, especially for Paula. When Paula did not know where to turn for help, a co-worker suggested that she approach her EAP for counselling to assist her in managing her stress and determining how to gain the co-operation and collaboration of her brother and sister.

The EAP counsellor's screening interview revealed that although Paula was distressed about her mother's impending death, she was much more distraught about the conduct of her two younger siblings. Both Andy and Margaret seemed to be oblivious to the reality that their mother was dying.

Neither could be encouraged by Paula to enter into a useful dialogue in order to attend to Louise's current needs, manage her declining weeks, or plan her funeral and burial. Paula's repeated requests for her siblings to endorse, openly refute, or discuss alternatives to Paula's proposals for their mother's care were either totally ignored or politely denied. Paula had become increasingly worried that Louise's care was being neglected.

After the first counselling session, Paula returned. She stated that the initial interaction with the counsellor had helped her recognize that her siblings' conduct was likely linked to their inability to deal with their mother's emotional pain, and to witness her gradual physical decline. Consequently, Paula decided to change her approach and empathize more, and be more gentle with her siblings. She let them know that she was also frightened and had found that she was frequently in tears as she watched her mother's health fail more each day. She told them that she felt very stressed and very isolated. Paula suggested that maybe a third party could help them communicate and work more effectively together. When she recommended that they accompany her to an EAP counselling session, they both agreed to attend.

When the counsellor became aware of Paula's request, he said he would comply, provided that individual meetings with Andy and Margaret were held in advance of any group interaction. These meetings explored their individual needs, interests, concerns, and hopes regarding the group interaction. The counsellor agreed that Paula's assessment of her siblings' willingness to participate in a mediated session was valid. Three informal mediation sessions followed during which the three siblings managed to discuss their misunderstandings and mutual anxiety, examine Paula's care plans and funeral arrangements, and determine how they could work together to cope with the weeks ahead.

After the three sessions, the siblings decided they could manage on their own. They mutually agreed that the mediator did not need to prepare a written agreement and all were appreciative of the mediator's offer to meet with the group again upon request in a follow-up session if needed. As the mediated discussions evolved and each person's understanding increased, Paula's anxiety declined markedly. Paula stated that the mediated sessions enabled her both to remain on the job at the institution where she was employed, and to decline her family physician's offer to provide anti-anxiety medications and a written request that she be excused from work for an unspecified period. A follow-up call several weeks later revealed that collaboration had continued and no further sessions were required. The entire process expended totaled six hours of successful EAP service delivery.

Family mediation: A formal marketed EAP service

When couples separate and the potential for a divorce arises, many counsellors, lawyers, and court systems endorse the formal process of family mediation. Due to the high level of skill and time allocation required, few EAPs can afford to include this service in regular contracts with employers. However, when the service is offered at fair market value, an EAP can provide employees and their partners with a readily accessible and potentially more affordable alternative to other providers offering this service.

Fundamental to family mediation is the need for role and task clarity, a concise contractual agreement, back-up lawyer support for each party, voluntary participation without threat or coercion, absence of any new legal initiative during the process, and freedom for any party to withdraw at any time. The freedom to stop the mediation and withdraw is especially important for the mediator, if the mediator believes that either party is using the mediation process to bully the other party or unreasonably extend or delay the proceedings. For instance, it is possible that one party may try to buy time to establish a status quo for custody purposes or complete a plan to conceal assets. One additional need is for the parties to understand that the mediator's final report that will be sent simultaneously to each party's lawyer as a formal *Memorandum of Understanding*; but that the Memorandum is not the formal legal Separation Agreement (Landau, Bartoletti, & Mesbur, 1997). The legal Separation Agreement is a totally separate document that follows; it is based on the *Memorandum* and is prepared for filing with the Family Court. This legal Separation Agreement is constructed by one party's lawyer and then reviewed prior to signing by the other party's lawyer, who ensures that it contains the details of the agreement described in the mediator's *Memorandum*. At the time of filing with the Family Court, the legal Separation Agreement may be accompanied by additional financial information, where required by the law. The mediator's *Memorandum* usually details resolved issues and may, in some instances, briefly mention unresolved issues as well. However, the mediator usually documents these unresolved issues separately and forwards them to each legal counsel simultaneously under separate cover. In some instances upon the request of each party the lawyers may collaborate, make recommendations, and suggest that the parties return to the mediator in order to re-examine and try again to resolve or reconcile these issues. The following case example highlights what may transpire in a family mediation.

Case Example: Sean and Debbie—Separating Couple
After 12 years of marriage, Sean, age 37, and Debbie, age 36, mutually decided that their differences could not be resolved. Couple therapy had

failed and a trial separation convinced them their marriage was over. They admitted that the well-being of their children had been the reason why they had tried so hard to save their marriage. They were committed to reaching a settlement that placed the needs of their children, Emily (age nine) and Mark (age seven), first. Following the decision to live permanently separate and apart, Sean and Debbie inquired about mediation through Sean's EAP. Contact with the EAP led to a conjoint exploration of mediation and the signing of a formal contract explaining the process and responsibilities of the mediator and of each party. It was agreed that mediation would include the development of a comprehensive parenting plan, a division of assets, a plan for child support, and an exploration of the need for spousal support. The family mediator then met individually with each party to clarify expectations, discuss concerns, and be assured that neither child nor spousal abuse nor any other serious problems were present to negate the role of mediation. The mediation process continued to a successful completion, in spite of the following concerns: the couple's agreement about the pick-up and drop-off times for the children when one parent took over from the other; the participation in child care by one relative; and the need to send out each party's pension statement to an actuary as recommended by one lawyer. The parties agreed that the mediation process was efficient and provided at minimal cost for time spent with the mediator, for the mediator's time to dialogue as needed with each legal counsel, and for documentation resulting in the mutually acceptable final *Memorandum of Understanding*.

Workplace Alternative Dispute Resolution (ADR): A formally marketed EAP service

Within the past two decades, Alternative Dispute Resolution has become an acceptable, economical, and desirable method of resolving serious conflicts between individuals, systems, and sub-systems within both the public and private sectors. This process, as in other types of mediation, enables disputing parties to share ownership of their mutual agreement to settle differences when participation is based on their interests and their needs. Decisions are reached without turning the decision-making over to a third party, who is acting as judge or arbitrator. When interacting persons or systems with differing values, goals, and objectives become conflicted, false assumptions about the other party are often made and may result in hostile and damaging actions. When each party is willing to negotiate and base a desire to settle differences on collaboration and relationship-building as opposed to power, rights, politics, territory, and possessiveness, ADR offers an effective route to resolution and reconciliation (Adams, 1994; Landau & Landau, 1999; Tannis, 1989; Wright, 1996).

In ADR, parties are encouraged to exchange information about their positions and then mutually define their problems in detail. This is followed by a collaborative exploration of potential alternative methods to resolve or reconcile differences, and the selection of the best mutually desirable alternatives or a "best alternative to a negotiated agreement" (BATNA). The process ends with a concise *Memorandum of Understanding* prepared by the mediator. This *Memorandum* usually contains mutually defined consequences, which will apply if the terms of the mediation agreement are breached—including how future deliberations will be funded (Landau & Landau, 1999; Wright, 1996).

Case Example: Zeb and Peter
Zeb, a 45-year-old pipe fitter, and Peter, a 39-year-old electrician, were required to work together in overhauling an extensive computerized plant sewage system at a large manufacturing site. Both men were long-term employees of a complex multinational corporation, and were highly respected skilled tradesmen with strong personalities. In the workplace, each worked in a separate department, was accountable to different supervisors, and belonged to different unions. Each man had also come from differing cultural backgrounds and despite their seniority, neither had encountered the other previously.

Zeb and Peter began to berate each other, subtly impede each other's work, and complain bitterly to their respective supervisors and union personnel about the other person's disposition and incompetence. Slowly their supervisors became aware of the seriousness of the conflict. They met and mutually decided to request a meeting with both men and their respective union stewards. This meeting began in a calm, matter-of-fact manner, but rapidly deteriorated into a heated argument and shouting match. All parties were clear that the conflict could not be resolved, and the matter was referred to higher levels. Eventually, the company's senior manager and the union president were individually apprised of the problem. The senior manager subsequently contacted the union president and suggested that due to the financial consequences and time constraints, mediation rather than arbitration would be the most effective and efficient route to resolving the problem. A joint management–union agreement was reached to mediate the dispute using an external third-party mediator. The company agreed to fund whatever was needed. The EAP was recognized as a reliable, independent provider of ADR services. The EAP was asked to participate and all parties agreed that the EAP mediator would conduct the

ADR deliberations at arm's length, involving only the two men in dispute. The ADR mediator would also be responsible for all preparatory details, including identification of a neutral site.

The EAP's designated ADR mediator passed all screening requirements, completed the necessary groundwork, and began conducting a closed ADR mediation. The process evolved rapidly. Within two three-hour sessions each party had agreed that neither wished to sabotage the mediation process; personality differences cited earlier were not a genuine root cause of the conflict; and the real problem between the two tradesmen was an inability to communicate with each other. Neither man had been briefed by his supervisor prior to beginning the job. Consequentially, neither man understood the other's mandate, roles, tasks, or the method selected to do the job. Neither had also been encouraged, or had been willing, to take the time to explain his personal expectations of how the work would be successfully completed. Mutual respect and collaboration generated through the ADR process resulted in an innovative agreement that was satisfactory to each. The details of the settlement were recorded in writing by the ADR mediator. These were subsequently reviewed, approved by both parties, and shared with management and union representatives.

Conclusion

The decision by EAPs to provide family and ADR mediation services requires caution. EAPs need to be very selective in recruiting their family-mediation and ADR professionals, and in determining which conflicts will be accepted for mediation. Both family and ADR mediators should be formally trained; thoroughly familiar with the nature and operations of the persons and systems requesting intervention; and be apprised of all policies, procedures, legal agreements, and other documents that may have an impact on the process. They must be willing to be screened by all parties involved, have the right to refuse to mediate, have access to the EAP's legal advisors if needed, and be in control of where, when, and how the mediation process will evolve.

Mediation, provided both informally and formally by EAPs, has earned recognition and respect as a potentially efficient and effective service for employees, their families, and their employers as well. When properly planned and delivered, mediation offers a viable, cost-effective alternative to more cumbersome and costly arbitrated and legislated processes. As an added bonus for disagreeing parties, it is based on their interests and needs as opposed to rights, keeps the decision-making process out of the hands of third parties, and enables the parties to be totally self-directed and in control of their own destiny.

Endnote

1. Folberg & Taylor, 1984; Baruch & Folger, 1994; Landau, Bartoletti, & Mesbur, 1997.

References

Adams, D. W. (1982). Terminally ill patients. In S.A. Yelaja (ed.), *Ethical issues in social work.* Springfield: C. C. Thomas.

Adams, G. W. (1994). *Mediation and the courts.* Toronto: Canadian Bar Association of Ontario.

Baruch, B. & Folger, J. (1994). *The promise of mediation: Responding to conflict through empowerment and recognition.* San Francisco: Jossey Bass.

Folberg, J. & Taylor, A. (1984). *Mediation: A comprehensive guide to resolving conflicts without litigation.* San Francisco: Jossey Bass.

Landau, B., Bartoletti, M., & Mesbur, R. (1997). *Family mediation handbook.* Toronto: Butterworths Canada.

Landau, B. & Landau, S. (1999). *Alternative Dispute Resolution: Mediation and negotiation skills.* Toronto: Co-operative Solutions.

Tannis, E.G. (1989). *Alternative Dispute Resolution that works.* North York: Captus Press.

Thompson, N. (2000). *Understanding social work: Preparing for practice.* London: MacMillan Press.

Timms, N. & Timms, R. (1977). *Perspectives in social work.* London: Routledge & Kegan Paul.

Wright, N. (1996). Principles of negotiation. In A. Stitt (ed.), *Alternative Dispute Resolution.* Toronto: C.C.H. Canadian.

Part IV

CASE STUDIES

The Challenge of Rural EAP:
The Iron Ore Company of Canada

Debbie Samson

Introduction

The following case study is an example of what one EAP practitioner has been able to accomplish, to enhance not only the wellness of workers employed by the organization and that of their families, but also the wellness of an entire community. This overview of one individual's practice, carried out with the support of a joint labour–management committee, illustrates that provision of an EAP is not only feasible in smaller and more isolated communities but also can become a centrepiece for developing broader community resources.

The Context

To claim that Labrador City, Newfoundland is situated in a "remote" location is something of an understatement. Located on the Labrador/Quebec border, it is a seven-hour drive, over mostly gravel road, from the nearest town of note, Baie Comeau, Quebec. To reach mainland Newfoundland takes a full two days: another seven-hour gravel-road trek to Goose Bay, followed by a 36-hour boat trip. Like so many communities that dot this region of Canada, the city boasts one major industry: mining. The Iron Ore Company of Canada (IOC) is the city's largest employer with nearly 1,800 workers on its payroll. These workers mine some of the world's finest iron ore, more than one billion metric tons of which have been unearthed since the inception of the Carol Project in 1962. IOC transports its products, both as concentrate and pellets, from Labrador City more than 400 kilometres by rail to a shipping terminal in Sept-Iles, Quebec.

Like employees from any workplace, at times IOC workers require assistance in meeting the personal problems that confront them. Relationship issues, parenting concerns, emotional or addiction problems—these and other problems of daily living can interfere with a worker's quality of life and job performance. For that reason, IOC established an Alcohol and Other Drug Addiction program in 1985. The program moved to a broadbrush format in 1991, at which time it came under the direction of a joint union–management committee. In that same year the organization received the Canadian Mental Health Association's prestigious Provincial Work and Well-Being Award for its efforts in developing this program for its employees. Currently, the day-to-day operations of the EAP are administered by a full-time internal coordinator under the guidance of the Joint Labour–Management Committee.

The community and workplace's remote location poses a special challenge for the EAP coordinator and committee. As Labrador City's population is not quite 8,000, there is not the same kind of continuum of health care and treatment services available as in larger Canadian communities. This has forced the EAP to be creative and, in some cases, to spearhead or establish new services that can meet client needs. In doing so the IOC EAP has become an integral part of the community's social-service network and health-care delivery system, benefiting not only the citizens of Labrador City but also those of the surrounding communities of Wabush and Fermont. In many respects, it is an "extreme" EAP, one that tests the limits of staff just as the extreme Canadian winters test the limits of its residents.

Service Provision

A variety of issues have been brought to the attention of the Iron Ore Company of Canada Employee Assistance Program and have been dealt with in both traditional and creative manners, as the following overview will illustrate.

  i)   Financial Issues
       In the early days of the program an unexpected number of employees came forward seeking EAP assistance due to financial concerns. Through program monitoring it was discovered that many workers who had not sought out assistance from the program for this reason could also benefit from learning basic money-management skills, such as how to develop a family budget. In response, the EAP sponsored a visit to Labrador City by a credit counsellor who held money-management workshops for both employees and the community at large. The workshops were so well attended that they have since been repeated on a regular basis.
 ii)   Alcohol and other Drug Addiction
       In the early 1990s, Labrador West, the towns of Labrador City and Wabush, had no ready access to services for those with alcohol or

other substance dependency issues. Individuals assessed as requiring inpatient treatment had to travel to other parts of Canada for care and assistance. To provide greater linkages and support, the EAP sponsored a visit by staff of a prominent treatment program. Several information sessions were held for both local health-care professionals and members of the community to provide education about the treatment process of addiction. Interestingly, a short time after the presentations, the Government of Newfoundland and Labrador opened a local office for Addiction Services.

iii) Critical Incident Debriefing Team
The EAP was instrumental in setting up the community's first critical-incident response team, the Labrador West Traumatic Event Defusing and Debriefing Team, in 1997. On the drawing board, it was initially conceptualized that such a team would benefit IOC workers. However, the EAP coordinator and committee quickly decided that the team should also be available to the entire community.

The IOC EAP coordinator facilitated meetings among community representatives to begin forming a broader team. With funding provided by the Iron Ore Company of Canada, the government and the community, specialists were again brought in to train team members. Almost immediately upon the training's completion, the Critical Incident Debriefing Team was called upon to perform several debriefings and defusings following incidents in the community. Afterwards, participants in the debriefings were asked to evaluate the services provided and almost uniformly rated the team "excellent," with a consensus that this type of service was long overdue in the area.

iv) Managing a Shiftwork Lifestyle
As shiftwork is a lifelong reality for many IOC employees, the EAP arranged for Jan Shearer, of the Canadian Institute for Shiftwork Studies, to travel to Labrador City to present a workshop on this topic. Shearer presented a very well-attended seminar on "Adapting to Shiftwork" and gave attendees a variety of tools to help them cope with this aspect of their working lives.

v) Menopause
In the late 1990s, as a number of spouses of employees were approaching their mid-40s, they contacted the EAP coordinator seeking information and help around the issue of menopause. The EAP, in conjunction with the local Public Health Office, developed and co-sponsored an information workshop on menopause, which was then offered to women in the general community who had

no affiliation or connection to the Iron Ore Company of Canada. Demand was so great and the response so positive that this has now become a regular offering of the Public Health Office.

vi) Eating Disorders

Over a brief period of time, the EAP received several requests to assist individuals with eating disorders. Again, as there was no local service providing support or assistance in this area, the IOC EAP arranged for a social worker specializing in this area and a representative of the self-help group Overeaters Anonymous (OA) to visit Labrador West. The two conducted a workshop for the general community and the employees and families of IOC entitled "Understanding and Planning for Personal Weight Control."

Following the workshop, several interested residents met with the OA representative and a local group was formed. The group continues to meet and has subsequently helped many people understand and overcome their eating-disorder issues.

vii) Child Abuse and Violence in the Family

On several occasions the EAP has co-sponsored child abuse and family violence workshops open to the entire community in concert with the Department of Human Resources and Employment, the Royal Newfoundland Constabulary, and other community agencies.

viii) Compulsive Gambling

Early in the 1990s, video gambling terminals (VDTs) were introduced in local businesses as a revenue-generating scheme for both the local establishments and the government of Newfoundland and Labrador. Not surprisingly, soon afterwards the EAP coordinator began fielding calls from workers with gambling problems, for which there was no counselling service available in the community (nor was there anyone in the larger community well versed in how to treat this impulse-control disorder). The EAP committee and coordinator researched the problem and decided to contact the Canadian Foundation on Compulsive Gambling. The EAP paid for a staff-person of the Foundation to travel to Labrador West to conduct public and professional workshops and seminars on compulsive gambling. As a direct result a Gambler's Anonymous chapter was formed to provide ongoing support in the community.

ix) Smoking Cessation

The EAP annually offers a four-week smoking cessation program for the general public. The EAP coordinator conducts the program, which includes presentations from a public health nurse, an addiction counsellor, a dietician and an instructor from the local fitness facility.

x) Stress-Management and Related Workshops

Through the program's ongoing monitoring process, and using the "self-reports" completed by clients as part of the EAP assistance process, it became apparent that workers at the IOC, like workers elsewhere, were experiencing increasing amounts of stress. This stress often manifested itself in the workplace, and was related to the difficult work performed by employees. In response, the EAP developed a one-day stress-management seminar to meet the expressed needs of the employees and their families. The success of this seminar has in turn led to the creation and presentation of additional sessions on anger, conflict, and assertiveness, which are now offered to employees, family members, and the entire community of Labrador West.

xi) Parenting

During their sessions with the internal program, many EAP clients described experiencing difficulties fulfilling their roles as parents. Working in a different capacity with the local child-protection committee, the EAP established an Active Parenting Program for all residents of Labrador West. A community committee was subsequently formed and individuals trained. This group has since taken over the training and continues to offer parenting programs throughout the community, and has the goal of expanding to offer a "Co-operative Parenting and Separation Program."

xii) Employee Support Programs

Many employees of the organization had over time, through no fault of their own, found themselves with insufficient financial means to get help for illness or disability. These situations were often brought to the attention of the local union executive, who felt that an Employee Support program was required. IOC employees and the company itself were both asked to contribute to a fund to help those in need. Employees voted to contribute the equivalent of one cent per hour worked to the Support Program, with the company matching that amount. The program provides assistance to employees and their dependents for "situations that arise due to extenuating circumstances." Upon inception, the Employee Support Program was placed in the hands of the EAP committee and coordinator to oversee and administer.

xiii) Shelter and Support for Men

From time to time men have come to the EAP to seek shelter and support when they and their children have been victims of violence within the family. Neither Labrador City nor Wabush has a shelter or safe house that will accept male clients. The EAP coordinator brought this to the attention of the general public, and a steering committee is currently researching options to meet this need identified by the EAP.

xiv) Grief and Loss

There is an element of loss in almost every problem that brings workers and family members to the EAP. For that reason, the EAP began holding a specific grief and loss workshop, "Windows: Healing and Helping through Loss." After learning of the initiative, the local hospital asked the EAP coordinator to conduct the workshop for its own intensive care staff, and like others, this workshop has been modified for presentation to the general community.

Conclusion

The mission of the Iron Ore Company of Canada's Employee Assistance Program, its Coordinator and Joint Union–Management Committee is to continuously meet the psychosocial needs of its workforce, as well as of those of the families of its employees, and whenever possible to assist the community at large. This Employee Assistance Program has moved from being merely a provider of brief intervention for employees and their family members to becoming a primary catalyst for social and health-care services in the community. The EAP has been responsible for both employee and community health-promotion activities, has sponsored speakers leading to the formation of self-help groups, and has been instrumental in the development of new services that otherwise might never have come into existence. Now that they do exist, these services meet a genuine need. This program demonstrates how EAP can create wellness not only in the workplace, but in the entire community; and it also reaffirms the responsibility employers have to create both a well workplace and a well community.

A Combined Internal/External Model:
The St. Joseph's Health Centre
Employee Counselling Service

Rick Csiernik, Brenda Atkinson, Rick Cooper,
Jan Devereux, Mary Young

Introduction

Since the 1960s, as a right of citizenship Canadians have had universal access to the full range of medical services offered by a complex and sophisticated hospital system. However, the 1990s witnessed unprecedented changes in the Canadian health-care sector, particularly in terms of how hospitals were funded and staffed. This produced a crisis in the delivery of health-care services. Deficit management became a priority for both federal and provincial governments. The shift from a health-care sector orientation to a health-care industry orientation in the Province of Ontario signified a paradigm shift that led to a re-allocation of resources, redesigned service delivery, restructuring of traditional roles, loss of employment, and a widespread sense of job insecurity. Despite threatened and actual job actions by physicians, nurses, and other health-care workers, massive organizational restructuring proceeded. This in turn led to unprecedented levels of stress for all health-care professionals: not only those who lost their jobs, but also those left behind to continue providing the historically expected levels of health-care services to individuals and communities with diminished resources. One resource that demonstrated itself to be of vital importance in supporting both individuals and organizations during this type of transition was the Employee Assistance Program (EAP).

St. Joseph's Health Centre and the Development of EAP

St. Joseph's Health Centre is situated in London, Ontario and is a recognized national and international centre of excellence in health care. The Sisters of St. Joseph, who came to London from Le Puy, France, founded the original St. Joseph's Hospital in 1888. Significant organizational changes began in 1984, when St. Joseph's Hospital (an acute-care facility with 530 beds) amalgamated with St. Mary's Hospital (a 184-bed chronic-care hospital) and with Marian Villa (a 247-bed home for the aged), thus creating the St. Joseph's Health Centre.

At the time of the merger, St. Joseph's Hospital had *Project Care*, an internal employee counselling service provided by staff of the hospital's Social Work Department. St. Mary's Hospital had a funded, external program provided by a community-based counselling agency, and Marian Villa had no official employee counselling program. The existing employee counselling programs at both St. Joseph's Hospital and St. Mary's Hospital were well utilized by employees with a high level of satisfaction, as evidenced by positive anecdotal feedback about the services being offered.

The amalgamation of the programs and departments in three health-care facilities was implemented over five years. In 1988 a task force with representation from all major employee groups, including senior management and union representatives, began to explore the feasibility of an integrated EAP. The advantages of each of the existing programs were outlined in conjunction with a review of various service-model options. Staff of the former St. Joseph's Hospital particularly valued their internal program for its convenience and accessibility, as well as for the fact that the counsellor was someone who was well acquainted with the organization. Staff of the former St. Mary's Hospital valued the off-site approach for its outside perspective and arm's-length relationship with the organization. Due to the perceived success of the previous programs, there was a strong desire by the task force not to lose what had already been working effectively and efficiently. Thus, in order to optimize the best of the two existing programs, a new integrated internal/external model was proposed—the St. Joseph's Health Centre Employee Counselling Service (ECS). The new model included an Advisory Committee, which met quarterly and which ensured communication regarding all aspects of program development, implementation, and evaluation. This approach was also intended as an indicator to staff of the newly formed St. Joseph's Health Centre that their ideas and needs were very important.

The St. Joseph's Health Centre Employee Counselling Services

The St. Joseph's Health Centre Employee Counselling Service began in January 1990 as a new and expanded program for all staff and family members living with them as well as physicians, volunteers, and retirees. The stated goal of the Employee Counselling Service was to provide a confidential, voluntary counselling service utilizing a short-term solution-focused counselling approach. The program brochure states that the Health Centre recognizes that "at some point most of us experience stress at work and in our personal lives which may affect our personal and physical health as well as our ability to be productive in our employment." The provision of a comprehensive counselling service, as an employee benefit, was one way that the institution demonstrated its ongoing concern for the physical, emotional, and spiritual well-being of its employees.

The ECS provided both on-site and off-site counselling options, each with a designated counsellor/coordinator. An external counselling service, WestBridge Associates Employee Assistance Services, was contracted to provide the off-site option. A counsellor with the St. Joseph's Health Centre Department of Social Work provided the on-site option. The counsellor/coordinators became responsible for the following:

- providing confidential assessments; individual, couple, family, and group counselling; and, if necessary, referrals to community agencies or other resources in the Health Centre or within the complement of psychologists, social workers, and other professional counsellors of WestBridge Associates;
- developing and delivering education, wellness, and outreach programs;
- administering a client/employee satisfaction survey at the conclusion of counselling;
- collecting and collating quarterly and year-end program statistics; and
- compiling an annual written report that included an evaluation of the previous year's service, and an outline of program goals and objectives for the next year.

Employees using the ECS had the choice of directly contacting the on-site internal counsellor/coordinator, located in a private location within St. Joseph's Health Centre, or the off-site external counsellor/coordinator at WestBridge Associates.

Integral to the success of ECS was the Advisory Committee. Established at the onset of the program, the ECS Advisory Committee closely monitored the program and its impact on employees. The fundamental structure of the Committee established in 1990 currently remains in operation. It is composed of representatives from all major employee groups, union and non-unionized, including a Vice-President. The internal/external counsellor/coordinators, the Coordinator of Occupational Health Services (who is responsible for the internal counsellor/coordinator) and a counsellor from the external provider, who is responsible for the external counsellor/coordinator, are also active members of the Advisory Committee. The ECS Advisory Committee is responsible for making recommendations for program development and changes, based upon a review of quarterly and annual statistics; they also are responsible for reviewing ECS policies, forms, and promotional materials. In addition, representatives of the various constituencies continuously reflect the impact on staff of ongoing hospital restructuring activities, and act as advocates for their member groups within the Committee.

ECS Program Evolution

When the new ECS program began in January 1990, there were 2,903 employees at the Health Centre. In the late 1980s it had become apparent that funding and staffing levels could not be maintained at existing levels, and that a new method of offering patient care would be necessary. In 1988 the first President and Chief Executive Officer who was not a Sister of St. Joseph was hired. He had a vision of the future of health care for the 1990s, and a mandate to lead St. Joseph's Health Centre into that future. It involved the introduction of Continuous Quality Improvement (CQI) which focused on establishing partnerships with "customers," use of data, and the demonstration of effective outcomes. In its first year of development, the ECS program responded with the introduction of a client satisfaction survey, as well as an increased awareness of, and service response to, the impact of change and stress on employees in the workplace.

In 1992 the first surge in program use was felt as the ECS experienced a 42.6 percent increase in the number of employees receiving service (Table 19.1). Not surprisingly, the ECS Advisory Committee was challenged to explore options for service delivery. The following year, the hospital restructuring/redesign process started, resulting in a shift from a departmental, hierarchical structure to a team-based, cross-functional structure. The ECS continued to be heavily used, with a 19.2 percent increase in caseload. In April 1993 counselling services ceased to be open-ended and a ten-session cap per referral was introduced. As well, counsellors were encouraged to develop a prioritized waiting list when necessary, and some prevention activities were temporarily curtailed.

As the St. Joseph's Health Centre underwent redesign and development of a new model of care, an Organizational Transition Team was established. The on-site ECS coordinator chaired a sub-committee for the team examining the emotional response to change by staff on both personal and professional levels. Although the global budget was decreased for the first time in 1994, the ECS was granted a budgetary supplement

Table 19.1: Financial and staffing changes compared with employee counselling services use (1)

Year	St. Joseph's Health Centre					Employee counselling services*	
	Funding		Employees		Telephone assessment and referral	In-office files/ cases	Total
1990	Global base			2903	26	153	179
1991	Increase	11.2%	Increase	4.1%	20	156	176
1992	Increase	9.2%	Decrease	2.8%	25	226	251
1993	Increase	2.2%	Decrease	1.3%	44	255	299
1994	Decrease	2.2%	Decrease	3.2%	34	210	244
1995	No change		Increase	0.7%	38	236	274
1996	Decrease	6.4%	Decrease	4.9%	32	275	307
1997	Decrease	6.2%	Decrease	4.1%	29	238	267
1998	No Change		Decrease	0.1%	32	230	262

* Does not include additional group work, outreach and wellness services provided to employees and family members

due to its increased focus on change and the provision of organizational change/transition-related group-work services to employees. In 1995 the ECS also shifted its reporting from the Department of Social Work to the Department of Occupational Health. While there were some initial concerns about the possible perceived association with Human Resources, the umbrella service under redesign for all staff-related services, there was no decrease in use of the ECS. As well, feedback from the client services surveys continued to be positive throughout this administrative transition. The increased funding for the ECS was maintained, demonstrating the commitment of the Health Centre's administrative team to support staff during this very stressful process.

In 1996 the Ontario Ministry of Health reduced by 6.4 percent funding to the Health Centre, leading to a reduction of nearly 5 percent in staffing and the implementation of organizational redesign. Job stress soon became the leading cause for seeking counselling. Due to budgeting constraints throughout the Health Centre, the ECS had its two-year supplemental funding discontinued. In a pro-active step, ECS counsellors were asked to participate in the design of the continuous employment program to aid employees to return to work in a timely fashion following short- or long-term absences from the workplace. In response to these events the ECS streamlined and computerized the collection of the intake-data form, and redesigned the client satisfaction survey in order to document the link between program utilization and specific indicators of improved job performance.

In 1997 the Ontario Ministry of Health reductions led to further staffing cuts. At the same time, the province of Ontario's Health Service Restructuring Commission (HSRC) proposed that the St. Joseph's Health Centre assume governance of Parkwood Hospital in London, a facility for chronic care and rehabilitation; and the recently amalgamated London/St. Thomas Psychiatric Hospital. While transfer of the governance of the psychiatric facilities was initially delayed, the governance of the Parkwood facility was assumed quickly. Parkwood Hospital had an external model of EAP service delivery, also using WestBridge Associates Employee Assistance Services. With a view toward integrating the existing Parkwood program with that utilized by the larger Health Centre, the programs at both sites underwent an analysis of their strengths, weaknesses, opportunities, and threats (SWOT). In 1998 the two separate Advisory Committees began holding joint meetings to develop a common vision and adopt a best-practices model of integrated and comprehensive employee assistance program delivery to begin in 1999.

Program Outcomes

Measuring outcomes of Employee Assistance Programs is a daunting and challenging task (Csiernik, 1995; 1998). The ECS has maintained statistics in a variety of areas since its inception. The Client Satisfaction Survey was reformatted in 1996 for implementation in 1997. Table 19.1 illustrates the change in caseload in the ECS since its inception in comparison with changes in funding and staffing.

In a comparison of ECS use in 1998 and 1990, it is interesting to note a 46-percent increase in the number of individual employees requesting assistance, despite nearly a 13-percent decrease in staff levels. The two years of highest usage—1993 (299) and 1996 (307)—coincided with significant organizational change and major anticipated or actual financial and staff reductions. It is important to note that between 1995 and 1996, the Health Centre had its budget cut by over 12 percent.

Likewise, there were significant changes in the problem profile between 1990 and 1998 (Tables 19.2a and 19.2b).[1] Presenting problems that have

Table 19.2a: Problem profile 1990–1996

	1990	1991	1992	1993	1994	1995	1996
Personal concern	65	42	76	60	54	59	62
Relationship issue	48	31	73	45	50	66	64
Marriage problem	41	45	60	55	36	44	54
Family difficulty	18	32	36	29	41	31	43
Violence	7	2	7	5	3	3	7
Child raising	8	6	8	13	9	7	20
Adolescent problems	8	8	12	12	19	12	22
Aging parents	4	2	0	3	4	1	1
Job stress	19	20	44	69	54	66	87
Financial difficulties	7	2	8	3	5	12	9
Grief and loss	12	5	8	7	15	17	12
Alcohol and drugs	6	4	12	2	8	9	1
Retirement	1	0	0	0	5	1	1
Other	4	0	0	0	1	6	1

Table 19.2b: Problem profile 1997-1998*

	1997	1998
Personal concerns	70	59
Family concerns	115	117
Violence	3	4
Work	47	48
Addiction	1	2
Other	1	2

* In 1997, the categories for Problem Profile were collapsed to six categories and recorded based upon the primary reason an individual sought counselling. Prior to 1997, multiple reasons were captured.

increased since the inception of the ECS include relationship issues, family difficulties, child raising, and adolescent issues. Some increases have occurred simply because more clients used the service, though areas such as aging parents, financial difficulties, grief and loss, and alcohol/drug use remained relatively stable. Less than 2 percent of all problems presented to the ECS since its inception have been alcohol- or drug-related. This is notable as chemical dependency is the issue most commonly associated with the original development of Employee Assistance Programs in the 1940s. In 1993 job stress became the single greatest reason that employees contacted the ECS, and has remained one of the most frequent reasons for requesting ECS assistance.

Table 19.3 summarizes the results of the client-satisfaction surveys from 1991 to 1998. As with much client-satisfaction data collected, response rates were moderate, ranging from 16.1 percent in 1998 to 49.4 percent in 1992 (Table 19.3a). Thus, there are limitations in extrapolating the results of Table 19.3 to all ECS users. Nevertheless, the 440 users who did respond were extremely satisfied with the service responsiveness of the ECS, which consisted of ease, timeliness, and convenience of making an appointment to see an on-site or off-site counsellor (Table 19.3b). There was exceptionally high agreement throughout the surveys that the counsellors, both internal and external, heard and were able to understand the concerns of the employees. As well, not only did respondents state that they would use the service again, if required, but they also almost unanimously stated that they would recommend the ECS to co-workers. Between 60 percent and 71 percent of respondents claimed that their situation had improved, while an even greater number (81 percent average over the eight years reported) answered that they were better able to manage their problem after meeting with the ECS counsellor.

The final section of the client-satisfaction questionnaire asked program users to comment upon the impact of counselling on their work performance. A significant majority in each year stated that counselling had led to an overall improvement in their work performance, ranging from 75 percent in 1994 to 100 percent in 1998. Over the eight-year period reported, an average of 40 percent of respondents stated they had improved concentration as a result of using the ECS; over 20 percent reported improved attendance at work; 37 percent reported improved relations with co-workers; 23 percent reported improved supervisory relationships (Table 19.3d); and 37 percent reported improved productivity. Overall, of those who replied, there was a strong belief that the Employee Counselling Service had been instrumental in improving their ability to work more collaboratively and effectively.

Conclusion

St. Joseph's Health Centre's commitment to a staff-focused approach to employee assistance programming was established early, with the initial decision to adopt an innovative service model designed to address the specific needs of staff in a merger situation. The positive outcomes of the resulting Employee Counselling Service highlight the importance of

Table 19.3: Client satisfaction survey responses

Table 19.3a: number of respondents

	1991	1992	1993	1994	1995	1996	1997
Total respondents	52	77	62	48	59	60	45
% of new cases	34.0	49.4	27.4	18.8	25.0	21.8	18.9

Table 19.3b: Service responsiveness

(Responsiveness defined as accessibility, timeliness, and convenience of appointments)

	1991	1992	1993	1994	1995	1996	1997
% satisfied	97	95	94	96	95	96	98

Table 19.3c: Client satisfaction with counselling process (%)

	1991	1992	1993	1994	1995	1996	1997
Counsellor understood my concerns	96	95	96	94	98	98	98
I was better able to manage my problem	69	88	71	68	80	82	98
My situation improved	63	71	69	60	69	71	*
I would use the ECS again	98	96	100	92	98	98	*
I would refer a co-worker to the ECS	96	99	100	98	100	100	*

* not asked

Table 19.3d: Impact of counselling on work performance

	1991	1992	1993	1994	1995	1996	1997
Increase in overall performance	77	77	84	75	94	85	100
Improved relations with co-workers	17	20	21	17	38	22	70
Improved relations with supervisors	8	10	15	28	22	10	37
Improved productivity	21	22	35	22	31	32	67
Improved attendance	10	9	13	14	22	13	33
Decreased stress	69	70	73	72	80	60	*
Improved concentration	37	46	37	42	40	45	*

* not asked

tailoring an EAP to be responsive to an organization's unique needs and the necessity of maintaining a pro-active employee counselling program.

The combined on-site/off-site model has proven to be an effective program design for the St. Joseph's Health Centre. The program design, along with regular communication between the on-site and off-site providers, ensures staff of the maximum benefits of choice. Even more fundamental to the success of the program, however, is the program's demonstrated flexibility and capacity to remain open to new information and ideas. A key success factor in the ability of the St. Joseph's Health Centre ECS to continue to respond to the profound changes experienced in the Canadian health-care sector during the 1990s has been its connection to the impact of those changes on staff/employees through a working Advisory Committee. Regular meetings/discussions through the Advisory Committee process have ensured continuous dialogue and enabled the ECS to identify and respond to employee needs as they arise within the context of continuous change.

In retrospect, St. Joseph's Health Centre of London has developed an Employee Counselling Service which equipped both program staff and its Advisory Committee members to deal with a process of integration and service development necessary for the ongoing evolution of the new and still-changing organization. As clinical programs move from and are added to St. Joseph's Health Centre, the ability of the ECS to adapt to each additional change will continue to be challenged. However, the ECS structure and processes created have placed the program in a position to effectively meet those challenges.[2]

Endnotes

1. In 1997 a new data-collection system was instituted that did not report problem profile in the same manner as the previous seven years.
2. In 2003, in response to the SARS concern within the Ontario health-care system, all employee counselling was moved off-site.

References

Csiernik, R. (1995). A review of research methods used to examine Employee Assistance Program delivery options. *Evaluation and Program Planning* 18(1), 25–36.

Csiernik, R. (1998). A profile of Canadian Employee Assistance Programs. *Employee Assistance Research Supplement* 2(1), 1–8.

Part V

CREATING WELLNESS

━━━━━━━━━━ **20** ━━━━━━━━━━

Spirituality and Work

David W. Adams and Rick Csiernik

> Who can separate his faith from his action, or his belief from his occupations?
>
> *The Prophet*, Kahlil Gibran (Knopf, 1965).

Case Studies

Barbara

Barbara, age 43, is a registered nurse with 10 years' experience in a large teaching hospital. She worked as an acute-care oncology nurse in the same unit for five years. Last fall, due to cutbacks in funding, she was moved to a surgical unit. Since then, she has struggled with her new assignment and encountered many frustrations. For example, the nurse assigned to orientate her to ward procedures was reluctant to provide detailed instructions, saying she was too busy. Being a newcomer, Barbara did not want to complain, so she kept silent. When she was ill with the flu in November and missed five working days, Barbara returned to her unit with trepidation. She knew whenever the ward was short her co-workers grumbled, and sometimes made it difficult for anyone who took additional time off. She was no exception, and on her first weekend she was left with the heaviest patients and a disproportionate workload compared to the "old regulars." When she fell behind in her work, she was left to fend for herself. At the end of the day, she was still trying to catch up while everyone else left on time. Two days later, the nurse manager told Barbara that she hoped Barbara would not make a habit of working late and taking time off ill. Barbara was upset. In her previous position, the health-care professionals worked as a team, helped each other, and took a positive approach to caring for patients and

257

their families. As a primary-care nurse and relief team leader, she had felt close to everyone. She was appalled that on her new unit several colleagues told her families were a "time-consuming pain," and that nurses were paid to do nursing care, and not to baby-sit. If patients or families had medical questions, they suggested that it was not the nurse's responsibility to answer them. Physicians and residents needed to earn their money for a change. They also told her not to worry about the nurse manager, as she didn't pay much attention to details on the unit since she was too busy elsewhere—the message was not to bother her or "stir up" her emotions.

Over Christmas and New Years, as usual the on-duty scheduling was done by one of the regular nurses on the unit. As the newcomers, Barbara and two other recently transferred nurses worked 12-hour shifts on days on Christmas, New Year's Eve, and New Year's Day. In early January, she was very fatigued, developed a severe migraine headache, and had to use two more sick days. On returning, Barbara felt very self-conscious and was certain two senior colleagues resented her absence and would likely hold it against her. As expected, she again received the heaviest workload.

On a Friday afternoon in late February, when Barbara's mother died suddenly due to a coronary, Barbara was due to work nights from 7 p.m. to 7 a.m. She was devastated by her mother's sudden death, but immediately worried that if she were off again her colleagues were certain to "punish" her. Her mother was buried Monday and reluctantly, Barbara was given Friday, Saturday, and Sunday as bereavement leave and Monday and Tuesday nights as her regular days off. On Saturday, the nurse manager called Barbara and coldly told her she had approved three days' bereavement leave and was sorry that her mother had died. No one from her new unit came to the funeral home or went to the funeral. When Barbara returned to work the day shift on Wednesday, only one nurse, the float social worker, and the area chaplain were consoling. In the middle of her first shift, Barbara started to cry and briefly left the area. One nurse offered to help by calling the nurse manager for relief, enabling Barbara to go home. The other nurses paid little attention. She thought she overheard one nurse say to the other, "What's the matter with her? By now she should be able to manage her feelings and get on with it."

Father Mark
Father Mark is a 35-year-old assistant chaplain and serves in a hospice, a nursing home, and a rural community hospital. As the living quarters for the clergy are located 17 miles away in the next community, Mark requested permission to rent a small apartment in the community where he works (he

is frequently on night call and has never liked driving, especially in winter). To his surprise, he was offered such accommodation by a local physician, free of charge.

In addition to his dislike of night driving, Mark has a mild residual limp resulting from a childhood disease. He readily suffers from extreme fatigue if physically overtaxed or sleep-deprived, but has hidden this from most of his peers given their their tendency to gossip and be critical. His supervising chaplain lives on church property in the next community and works within walking distance of the large teaching hospital. He and several other male clergy who live in the same residence cannot understand Mark's request. They have been upset and have been avoiding him as much as possible. Only the housekeeper and cook are currently speaking to him.

Due to Mark's desire to be more independent and have his own parish, he is fearful of short-circuiting his supervisor; and from previous discussions, knows that if he approaches the Bishop, he may be rapidly reassigned to a less desirable posting. For Mark it is not the hospice, nursing home, or hospital that are challenging his wellness; it is those directly in charge of his career, his work assignment, and his living conditions.

Kathy

Kathy (age 25) is a quiet, intelligent, and creative physiotherapist. Last summer she took special courses and rapidly learned new skills prior to joining a private clinic employing 14 other physiotherapists. From the beginning, the clinical director was ecstatic about Kathy's skills and enthusiasm. She immediately assigned her to a special unit to work with practitioners from several other disciplines in a large rehabilitative facility.

After three weeks, Kathy was shocked to learn that:

- her skills were devalued;
- referrals seldom came her way despite obvious patient need;
- several staff constantly made unsavoury comments about the patients, physicians, social worker, and nutritionist;
- the clinical director was seldom present and leadership was generally lacking; and
- relatives were expected to be the major care providers and were openly criticized for their omissions or questions.

Kathy's new skills were totally lost. She found herself becoming increasingly irritable and less interested in her job. Her next step seemed to be to request a transfer or resign her position.

The Seven Challenges of the Workplace

In contemplating the difficulties faced in these three cases, we can increase our understanding of the stressors faced by each professional by delineating seven challenges that impact their daily working lives:

i)   the practical: how can Barbara deal with the disproportionately heavy workload for which she is responsible?

ii) the physical: how can Father Mark continue to cope and manage his physical fatigue?

iii) the behavioural: how can Kathy maintain her professional manner and practice effectively when others behave so negatively, and from Kathy's perspective, so destructively?

iv) the emotional: how can Barbara manage her grief in such a demanding and hostile work environment?

v)   the cognitive: how can Father Mark, in his current situation, strategize to effectively meet the demands of the different organizations that he serves and fulfil the needs of his diverse clients?

vi) the social: how can Kathy talk openly, associate with co-workers, and become part of a health-care team when she knows she is disliked as much as other professionals and her skills and abilities are not valued?

vii) the spiritual: how can Barbara, Mark, and Kathy maintain their spiritual wellness when faced with increasingly negative work environments?

These seven areas are typical of the regular challenges faced by Employee Assistance professionals; they are also typical of the challenges that we personally encounter regularly in our workplaces. They are not only the source of our stresses and frustrations, but also the forces that involve and motivate us. They are simultaneously the obstacles that prevent us and our clients from acquiring and maintaining a level of wellness, while also being the foundations of our wellness that provide us with a sense of achievement and feelings of success and wholeness (Csiernik, 1995).

Of these seven aspects of workplace wellness, spirituality is the most recent to be actively studied (Adams & Csiernik, 2001; 2003). The idea of spirituality at work raises its own profound questions. Does a workplace have a sense of spirituality? If so, is this simply the cumulating of the spirituality of individual workers or is it a gestalt, with workplace spirituality being greater than the individual spirituality of each employee? What does the spirit of the workplace look like? What are its components? What are the qualities of working life that prevail in an environment that has little or no spiritual dimension?

Spirituality and the Workplace

Spirituality includes a person's ability to transcend the physical limits of time and space, the ability to reason, to will, to be creative, and to seek meaning. Spirituality also entails being self-aware, adhering to values, being ethical, being connected with others, and maintaining a belief system that includes a religious dimension (Morgan, 1993). Spirituality hinges on three critical assumptions:

i)   an awareness of the existence of a supreme power or force;
ii) the innate yearning of people for connection with this supreme entity; and,
iii) the belief that this power is interested in humans and acts upon this relationship in order to promote changes that benefit humans (Anderson & Worthen, 1997).

If these assumptions are correct, how does the supreme power, how does God, impact our work environments and influence change in the workplace? Are contemporary workplaces aware of such assumptions, or indeed aware of any aspects of spirituality? Are they capable of meeting any of the spiritual needs of individuals, let alone all of them? Has the typical workplace not, in fact, been antithetical to meeting individual spiritual needs and historically been a force that prevents us from reaching spiritual fulfilment? Does God as the supreme power really impact our work environments and influence change in the workplace?

In comparing the spiritual components of the individual and those of the workplace, one finds similarities with respect to dynamics, responsiveness to stimuli, the capacity to reason, the endorsement of values and ethics, creativity, and the ability to transcend individualism (Adams, 2000). When we contemplate the components of spirituality, we find that workplaces, like people, tend to be governed on some level by principles that are based on a system of values and a code of ethics. Such principles have an extensive and diverse sphere of influence and may define how to attend to their product, be it treating families or disposing of hazardous waste. At the same time each workplace is faced with the need to demonstrate creativity and remain innovative in order to compete and survive in this continuing time of rapid institutional and technological change.

Further spiritual comparisons between individuals and workplaces tend to reflect more differences than similarities. For example, workplaces are created by individuals rather than being ontological. They seek meaning in a systemic as opposed to a personal context, and in most instances, lack a religious dimension, and certainly do not transcend an earthly presence. However, one other critical similarity should be noted. Just as individuals are vulnerable and may fear death, contemporary workplaces are vulnerable to failure and dissolution, a reality to which anyone who has experienced a plant closure can readily attest (Table 20.1).

Table 20.1: A spiritual comparison

Individual	Workplace
Living	Dynamic
Sensate	Responsive to stimuli
Reasoning	Learning and strategizing
Valuing	Valuing
Ethical	Ethical
Rational thinking	Governed by reason
Creative	Creative
Individual	Transcends individualism
Fears dying	Fears dissolution
Seeks meaning	Seeks place within a system(s)
Religious	Religion not a factor
Ontological	Created by individuals
Transcends life on earth	Earthly

Six Stations of our Spiritual Journey

Percy's (1997) conceptualization of the spiritual journeys taken by both individuals and workplaces allows us to further examine the fit between the spiritual needs of ourselves and the workplace. Percy describes six stations or stages of our inner spiritual journey: innocence, independence, institution, irritation, insight, and integration. We suggest that these six specific stages are readily applicable to our working lives. The first station, *innocence*, is the birthplace of hope. It is based upon trust and a belief that there is justice in the workplace environment that we are entering when we are hired by an organization. The second station, *independence*, revolves around the ideas and ideals of determining who we are, where and how we fit into this new setting, and how we strive to be creative and self-sufficient. If we are successful, the outcome of independence is to become the masters of our own fate. The third spiritual station is *institution*. Here, as individuals we are pressured to conform, to meet the standards and norms of others, and to fit into a cultural box. The workplace is among the most prominent and dominant of institutions in our society (Morgan, 1986). It can be a controlling force that may eventually both overpower and disempower us, as witnessed in our three case studies. Too often, as individuals we become stuck and cannot move beyond this stage in our spiritual journey, either in our personal lives or in the workplace.

The next station of our spiritual evolution, *irritation*, is perhaps the most essential and difficult stage to move through in order to continue moving toward spiritual wellness. Here, we actively seek our own destiny and rebel against the power others hold over us, especially the power of institutions and the workplace. In order to move forward, we must successfully resist external controls and achieve self-direction. It is often during this re-emergence of youthful rebellion in the face of controlling forces that the real truth of corporate reality is perceived. We see how our individuality is curbed and our creativity limited. We frequently react with anger, and if we successfully emerge from this corporate dominance, we advance to the stage of *insight*. Here, we allow ourselves to be driven by our spirit. We shed what is unimportant and our power emanates from our soul. In the workplace, this stage involves a return to hope and a wisdom, born from revisiting the "why" of existence and examining how it conforms with our working self.

The last stage of our inner journey and our corporate journey is *integration*. In this stage we learn to truly value ourselves for our uniqueness; and it is here that we may reach Percy's (1997) spiritually better and deeper place. When we reach this place in our working lives we reach a place of harmony where our sense of self and purpose is integrated with our vocation. Unfortunately many of us are unable to experience the benefits of this stage, especially when we are employed by corporations characterised by an historic lack of spiritual wellness. We are limited in our ability to feel energized, valued, and fulfilled. Such environments support a belief that spirituality has a minimal impact on our work, and that spirituality does not belong in the workplace unless it is formally sanctioned or mandated.

Returning to the work environments of Barbara, Mark, and Kathy, we see that several spiritually unhealthy workplace characteristics are evident. These include unresolved conflicts, a lack of caring for people, continuous criticism, an endless flow of demanding tasks, "top down" and "absentee" management, a lack of recognition and respect, threats of dissolution or expulsion, a poor physical environment, and discrimination, both real and perceived. Each employee is confronted with workplace systems and sub-systems that are rejecting, demoralizing, and noxious. Each workplace contains the dominant and disempowering qualities that may force individuals to be anxiety-ridden and spiritually demoralised. Their progress along their spiritual journey is thwarted by organizations that stagnate and are unable to move forward on their own corporate spiritual journey. As well as creating spiritual turmoil, these workplaces perpetuate physical, emotional, and social pain that results in genuine suffering.

Managing and Overcoming Suffering in the Workplace

Historically, a key function of a strong spiritual self has been to enable us to effectively face, cope with, and overcome our personal and collective suffering (Maes, 1990). Our spirituality is essential to our belief that our suffering will be removed, or that we will be rewarded or compensated in some tangible manner for the suffering that we have endured (Epstein, 1994; Frankl, 1984; Maes, 1990). Our spirituality provides us with hope, connects us with forces beyond the present, gives us inner strength to cope, encourages us to look for meaning in our tribulations, and aids us in managing our lives and transcending our suffering (Eaton, 1988; Highfield, 1992). "Shuddering," the process of living through the pain and experience of our suffering, is a critical concept to consider when examining spirituality in the workplace. Shuddering occurs when we succumb temporarily to our suffering as we are caught up in the rapids of change in our daily and working lives and react to the cumulative stress and overload. The process of shuddering in the workplace draws upon, and may deplete, our spiritual strength (Percy, 1997). However, alternatively, it may enhance our spiritual energy and motivate us to regain control, find new hope and new purpose in our working lives, and move through the third spiritual development station of "institution," and on to the next stations of "irritation" and "insight." In the process of shuddering, we learn that we can and will use our renewed energy to move forward.

Spirituality is essential to being able to find faith in ourselves, in our beliefs, and in our connections to others. It is also vital in aiding us to find faith in an uncertain future. Shudderings are truly transitional points. These provide us with unique insights and even enlightenment concerning our states of being. As a result of shuddering, we may find the motivation, strength, and courage to make decisions such as staying in a spiritually unhealthy workplace, applying for a position of leadership, and trying to positively influence change in spite of the uncertainty. Contrarily, a shuddering may enable one to take the steps necessary to leave the workplace on one's own terms. Shuddering enables us to take risks that demonstrate initiative, creativity, and innovation, as we challenge stagnation or unhealthy or unreasonable changes. At the same time, shuddering may provide us with the impetus to reorder our work and family priorities, deal with personal life-cycle crises, or take action against unresponsive systems with, or on behalf of, our clients.

Spirituality: An Integral Component in Managing Workplace Challenges

Spirituality in the workplace is not only one of the seven challenges of working life, but it is also an integral component of all of the other challenges. Spirituality may provide the calm for us to find that we have the tools in place to deal successfully with the *practical challenges* of the workplace. It may assist us in coping with the *physical challenges* through encouraging self-care and the ability to balance the demands placed upon our physical selves. Spirituality may also contribute to meeting *intellectual challenges* by allowing room for humour and mutual support, particularly when we must manage demands emanating from a multitude of workplace stressors. *Behaviourally*, spirituality may motivate us to care for and respect each other, and perhaps move towards shared responsibility or ownership of the workplace as we engage in participatory democracy, and the sharing of common tasks. Spirituality may also provide respite, positive social interaction, and diversion in order to help us deal with the *social challenges* of the workplace. In summary, spirituality may bring to our working lives serenity, energy, direction, creativity, connectedness, goal attainment, and, perhaps most importantly, hope for the future. In reality, it is an essential force within the workplace and, as illustrated in Figure 20.1, can be viewed as the overriding factor that allows us to successfully meet all the challenges we encounter within the workplace.

Figure 20.1: Spirituality as an overriding force in meeting workplace challenges

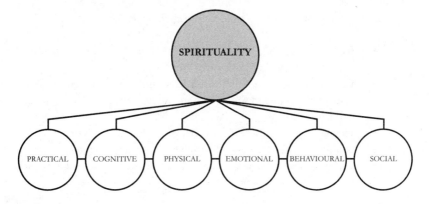

In a study of 154 helping professionals, social workers and nurses reported that their workplaces were the most stressful; by contrast, clergy (and those working in pastoral care) reported the least stress. Persons working in funeral homes and churches reported that the stress of their work resulted in the most significant negative impact on their spirituality. More importantly, however, it was found that those helping professionals with the greatest individual sense of spirituality were the most likely to state that their workplace had a positive emotional climate and produced less stress. A strong sense of personal spirituality appeared to contribute to wellness and assisted in counteracting workplace stress (Csiernik & Admas, 2002).

However, the obstacles to applying spiritual principles to the workplace are many and formidable. Fixed beliefs, chronic inaction, tolerance of employee abuse and neglect, culture dicta, economic deficiencies, emotional overload, social isolation, third-party forces, the unrelenting flow of information and demands created by the continually enhanced ability to communicate, and the lack of access to counsellors are all factors which may limit the spiritual growth and development of the workplace and everyone associated with it, including ourselves.

Toward a Spiritually Healthy Workplace

The keys to formulating and maintaining a spiritually healthy workplace are to be found in an organization's ability to be responsive to human needs, to engage people in planning and managing their working lives, and to find ways to enhance how employees feel about themselves, about their contribution to the workplace and its clientele, and about the workplace itself. If we return to the difficulties encountered by Barbara, Mark, and Kathy, we can recognise that in order to promote their spiritual well-being within the workplace some fundamental needs must be fulfilled. The following spiritual qualities would help each individual case:

- feeling acknowledged and valued for their skills, capabilities, and contributions to the workplace;
- being given help to gain the knowledge and skills required to engage both the system and their colleagues in supporting them personally and professionally;
- feeling respected for their knowledge, skills, and experience;
- feeling trusted to manage themselves and their jobs effectively;
- engaging with motivated colleagues in providing a unified approach to improving their working lives; and

- finding acceptance as a person with individual needs, concerns, and capabilities.

We can also suggest that for this to happen the workplace must be:

- dynamic and responsive to the needs of employees, the organization itself, and its clientele;
- prepared to acted efficiently and effectively at any time;
- able to manage and resolve conflicts and differences in order to achieve internal harmony;
- connected to external systems that may benefit the organization at large, the workplace, and the personnel within it;
- willing to take pride in its self-image and enable employees to do likewise, both for themselves and the workplace;
- able to promote and maintain an environment in which employees feel needed, respected, and valued by the employer and by each other;
- engaged in continuous evaluation of the human, as well as the business, component of the workplace;
- capable of measuring, acknowledging, and communicating success in human as well as business achievements to individuals and groups within the workplace and beyond;
- combining the acknowledgement of success, the need to continuously improve, and initiatives to resolve conflicts in order to stimulate personal motivation and promote teamwork; and,
- concerned about and tangibly engaged in promoting the health and well-being of employees, their families, their clientele, and the community at large (Table 20.2).

Conclusion

There is still much to study and learn about spirituality in the workplace. Work environments offer an exciting forum for exploration, creation, and innovation, as we strive to understand in greater detail the spiritual evolution of people and organizations. We have examined Percy's six stations of our inner spiritual journey, and their application to the workplace; and we have explored how spiritually unhealthy workplaces inhibit spiritual development and inflict spiritual suffering on their employees. In so doing we have taken advantage of Percy's creative term "shuddering" as it applies to the ability of each of us to experience and move through suffering, as we proceed along a continuum of spiritual development in the workplace. We have also discussed how spirituality is both an integral and overriding force influencing the other six workplace challenges and our ability to

Table 20.2: Spiritual wellness

Individual	Workplace
Alive/energetic	Dynamic/responsive
Feels capable	System ready to perform
Internal harmony	Internal harmony
Symptom-free	Conflicts managed
Externally connected	Externally connected
Functions effectively	Functions effectively
Positive self-image	Positive reputation
Positive mood	Positive work environment
Satisfied	Continuous quality improvement: always seeking positive workplace change
Able to enjoy	Measures and acknowledges success
Feels connected	Enables teamwork
Excited about life potential	Excited about future goal attainment
Values higher purpose	Values altruism/employees/clients

master them successfully. Finally, we have suggested how organizations can enhance the spiritual health of the workplace, its employees, and other people and systems affected by it.

In closing, we offer a definition of workplace spirituality to assist with the fostering of spiritually healthy workplaces beyond that discussed in chapter 1:

Workplace spirituality involves positively sharing, valuing, caring, respecting, acknowledging, and connecting the talents and energies of people in meaningful goal-directed behaviour that enables them to belong, be creative, be personally fulfilled, and take ownership in their combined destiny.

References

Adams, D.W. (2000). Seeking the lost spirit: Our quest for spiritual renewal in the workplace. *18th International Conference on Death, Dying, and Bereavement: Attending to the spiritual needs of the dying and bereaved.* Kings College, London, Ontario, Canada.

Adams, D.W. & Csiernik, R. (2001). A beginning examination of the spirituality of health care practitioners. In R. Gilbert (ed.), *Health care and spirituality: Listening, assessing, caring.* Amityville: Baywood.

Adams, D.W. & Csiernik, R. (2003). An exploratory study of the spirituality of clergy as compared with healthcare professionals. in G. Cox, R. Bendiksen & R. Stevenson (eds.), *Making sense of death: Spiritual, pastoral and personal aspects of needs, death, dying and bereavement*. Amityville: Baywood.

Anderson, D.A. & Wortham, D. (1997). Exploring a fourth dimension: Spirituality as a resource for the couple therapist. *Journal of Marital and Family Therapy* 23(1), 2–12.

Csiernik, R. (1995). Wellness, work and Employee Assistance Programming. *Employee Assistance Quarterly* 11(2), 1–12.

Csiernik, R. & Adams, D.W. (2002). Spirituality, stress and work. *Employee Assistance Quarterly* 18(2), 29–37.

Eaton, S. (1988). Spiritual care: The software of life. *Journal of Palliative Care* 4 (1/2), 94–97.

Epstein, D.M. (1994). *The 12 stages of healing: A network approach to wholeness*. San Raphael: Amber-Allen.

Frankl, V. (1984). *Man's search for meaning*. Washington, DC: Washington Square Press.

Highfield, M.F. (1992). The spiritual health of oncology patients: Nurses' and patients' perspectives. *Cancer Nursing* 15 (1), 1–8.

Knopt, A. (1965). *K. Gibran: The prophet*. New York: Basic Books.

Maes, J.L. (1990). *Suffering: A caregiver's guide*. Nashville: Abingdon Press.

Morgan, G. (1986). *Images of organizations*. Beverly Hills: Sage.

Morgan, J.D. (1993). The existential quest for meaning. In K. Doka & J.D. Morgan (eds.), *Death and spirituality*. Amityville: Baywood.

Percy, I. (1997). *Going deep in life and leadership*. Toronto: MacMillan.

21

A First Nations' Perspective on Work, the Workplace, and Wellness

Kelly Brownbill

> The Indian world was devoted to living;
> the European world to getting.
> Sequichie Hifler (1996)

Historical Perspective

In any examination of the difficulties of Canada's First Nations people succeeding in the mainstream workforce, it is important to consider the legacy of the past 500 years. The mechanics of contact between the original people of this land and the visitors from Europe are mirrored today in the struggle of First Nations people to thrive in the corporate world. Although there are numerous cultures among the indigenous peoples, some generalizations may nevertheless be made.

Prior to contact with European races, the society of First Nations people looked very different. Theirs was a world of harmony with nature, in which humanity was but one part of Creation. Human beings were not elevated to special status above other forms of life, but were in equal partnership with all that lived on Mother Earth. All things had a spirit, from the rocks and trees to animals, birds, and fish. So close was the tie between the natural world that First Nations people enjoyed a kinship with Creation that carried as far as their method of government.

Ancient teachings in many of the cultures indigenous to Canada describe stewardship of the land as a responsibility of the people. This concept of ownership of land was quite different from that of those communities who first came into conflict with settlers. The aboriginal perspective towards the land was more akin to the way we view children; we do not own our children, yet they belong to us. First Nations people did not own the land for their own exploitation; rather it was a gift from the Creator. That gift included with it the responsibility of caring for the land and all those who made their home on her. Combine this with the understanding that every time you cut down a tree you killed a brother, and it is easy to understand why the conflict between First Nations cultures and European settlers was inevitable: the aboriginal outlook was in distinct contrast to the Europeans' objectives.

Opposing views with the prevalent systems of government also made peaceful co-existence next to impossible. The norm in First Nations governments was a process of hereditary selection and consensus. Leaders truly governed for the people, and decisions were not made until all those who wished to do so had voiced their opinion. The clan system recognized then, as it still does today, different strengths in different people; therefore it may not have been clear to the Europeans at the time which individual "spoke" for the village. Different clan leaders would be sent to speak on their areas of expertise. Leaders were also not elevated to a higher status, but merely fulfilled their responsibility to the community in the same manner as all members. Any hierarchical structures would have been completely foreign to many of the cultures present before contact.

The power structure in Europe was based on the ownership of land and belongings as much as on an elevated position in a rigid, hierarchical class structure. In traditional ceremonies of First Nations people, "give-aways," the passing on your most prized possessions to others, ensured a distribution of wealth. The person with the biggest lodge had the biggest family. The concept of "owning" was more aptly described as "carrying," in the sense that aboriginal society believed all possessions were theirs only as long as the spirits willed it; giving away even the most treasured item was a certainty. Power based on acquisition was not the norm in traditional aboriginal communities.

This basic dichotomy created a downward spiral in the relationship between Europeans and Canada's First Nations peoples. From legislation such as the Indian Act to residential schools and the "Sixties Scoop," the term given to the proportionately higher percentage of native children removed from their homes and placed in foster care, the government set out to systematically assimilate these distinct societies. Beyond the incredible changes this wrought in communities and nations, it left a legacy that still haunts aboriginal people today. In recent history, First Nations people have had little or no control over their lives. Travel off reserve required a pass signed by a government official. Election codes were set by the Indian Act, and band council meetings were presided over by the Indian Agent. First Nations women who lost their status upon marrying a non-native man were no longer considered members of their community, and in many cases were not allowed to live on reserve. The Government of Canada literally controlled every aspect of aboriginal peoples' lives.

This period of struggle has left a daunting legacy. Many First Nations people today have never been taught the mechanics of choice. Although some may recognize that the choices they make have a direct influence on their lives, they have no process to utilize for assessing options. It is only recently—as change and progress have begun to halt the process of assimilation—that aboriginal youth can look to successful individuals in their communities, individuals who model that process of healthy choice.

Cultural Perspective

The Medicine Wheel is used by many of the indigenous cultures of North America as a guide to wellness. It is basically a tool, a gift from the Creator, which includes all the lessons needed to live a healthy, productive life. A Medicine Wheel is always a circle divided into four equal parts. The significance and teachings surrounding those four sections of the wheel vary depending on use; they may be the Four Directions, the Four Sacred Medicines, or the Four Aspects of Man, to name but a few. Included are the teachings of the Four Colours of Man. It is taught that the Creator made four different races of man, each with its own colour: a Yellow Race, a Red Race, a Black Race, and a White Race. The Creator gave each "Colour of Man" its own original instructions, its own place on the Earth to live, and a gift. Each colour of man received a different gift or ability, which set it apart from the other races. Each race could use this gift to better its members' lives and solve problems. Although each gift was powerful in its own right, it was only one of four abilities valuable to human beings. Ancient prophecies have been passed down throughout the generations, describing a time when all four Colours of Man would come to live on the ancient land of the First Peoples. The White Race, with its gift of movement, would be the first to arrive; but there would come a time when Turtle Island, the continent of North America, would be home to all races. At that time, the struggle would be to lay aside any differences, and combine all gifts for the good of everyone.

These teachings contain a premise not always found in other cultures and spiritualities. Certainly the first missionaries to come to this land believed that theirs was the only true path to salvation, and that they would be doing the indigenous people a true disservice if they did not show them the way. Yet many First Nations cultures believe not only that there are many different ways, but also that that is how it is supposed to be. Converting a person to a different belief system went against the teachings of the Medicine Wheel. The Creator gave each colour of man its own instructions; why would anyone change that?

Those First Nations people who were raised with traditional values, whether through ceremony or not, have a distinct view on cultural diversity. It is celebrated as the correct order of Creation, not as a challenge or obstacle to be overcome. The opposing view of most Christian faiths at the time was that theirs was the one true path to salvation. The vast divergence in belief, coupled with numerous other societal factors, made the attempt at assimilation inevitable. It was the unshakeable conviction of European religious leaders that they had to convert the natives to save them.

This led to an almost complete destruction of traditional First Nations spirituality. The Residential School System converted aboriginal children to Christianity at an alarming rate. In addition, there was a national outlawing of aboriginal ceremony and cultural practices. The path back is twisted and incomplete; many native people in Canada today are following traditional lifestyles as closely as they can, while others attempt to combine aboriginal ceremonies with deeply entrenched Christian beliefs. The struggle to retain the culture and spirituality is not only a personal quest, but is also imperative to the preservation for future generations.

It is important to recognize, however, that the majority of First Nations peoples in Canada may not have a link to their traditions. Even without adding different cultures into the equation, First Nations communities can be divided over issues of religion and spirituality, Christians versus traditionalists, Catholics versus Protestants. The conflict continues to disrupt the health of aboriginal communities.

The Significance of Choice

One of the skills required to successfully negotiate the modern-day workplace is the ability to choose. Although employees today are faced with many circumstances over which they have no control, each day at work includes numerous opportunities for choice. Punching the time clock, adhering to policies and procedures, even showing up for work are all a matter of choice for an individual. Hopefully, by the time most adults reach the workplace, they have some understanding that their actions control their destiny.

First Nations people have often had difficulty with the ability to chose. Historically much of the freedom of choice was removed from their existence through government control. The Indian Act still controls the election process on most reserves in Canada. Funding from the government, except in very rare cases, continues to flow regardless of the actions or behaviours of a community. A typical 40-year-old First Nations individual raised on a reserve in Canada may not have had the chance to determine his or her own destiny through personal choice; the options needed to exercise choice were unavailable.

As a result of historically fewer and limited mainstream employment opportunities available to First Nations people, on average, many First Nations employees who enter a mainstream workplace have little if any employment experience. Many small or family-run businesses, the most common type of business found on reservations, have few if any formal performance standards. One prominent example is the limited use of written or rigidly enforced attendance policies. This leaves an employee unprepared to choose between coming to work, or facing the consequences of a company-wide policy. Quite often, First Nations employees working in a large corporation for the first time are surprised at the outcomes of choices they have made. More than one aboriginal employee has found themselves terminated as a result of poor attendance. Often, they are baffled at the outcome, as they have a legitimate reason for the last absence. They fail to see that the poor choices of the previous absences are the real reason for dismissal, not just the final occurrence.

As well, the choice of employment opportunities has been significantly reduced for aboriginal people in Canada. Isolated locations, poor education, and a societal, even systemic, governmental belief in the inferiority of First Nations people have created a number of barriers to entering the workforce. Non-native Canadians can usually look to past generations for guidance in surviving a working environment; however, aboriginal people have significantly fewer role models. In some of the more isolated First Nations, families are only one generation away from traditional methods of existence, which involved very limited contact outside of their community.

Even an understanding of corporate structure can be foreign to aboriginal people when they join the workforce. The modern-day employer expects from his or her employees a level of sophistication or understanding of hierarchy, which is missing in many First Nations situations. The hierarchy of a workplace or even a government can be foreign to aboriginal people raised in a small, close-knit community. Traditionally, chiefs and leaders were not considered to be of greater status than community members; rather, their gifts were recognized as being well suited to the task of leadership. Everyone in a community would have their own gifts, and be recognized for them, rather than a few individuals being revered because of the position they had achieved. Leaders led the community from a shared vision; consultation with elders and community members was the norm in the decision-making process of a traditional aboriginal community. This is very unlike the usual North American workplace.

As the ability to choose slowly eroded, so too did the community structure. Family and community were central to traditional First Nations life. Societal norms and government processes were family-focused. The culture was so involved in family and community that the concept even embraced the world around them: all Creation was family. In today's environment, family structure is still central to society, and can look quite different from a nuclear family. Given the severe social and economic challenges on reserves, many First Nations people were raised by extended family members, or even community members with no blood relation. Legal proceedings such as adoptions were not the norm; the needs of children had priority over formalizing the relationship.

A sense of community is still very important to First Nations people. When removed from their communities and placed in a corporate setting, they will make a community around them. Relationships at work tend to come out of balance as they look to their co-workers to provide the feelings of safety and belonging—core components of wellness necessary for a community setting. This can, however, also escalate into destructive behaviours. Joining "the guys" from work for a drink at the end of the day can easily be used as a replacement for a healthier support system. Aboriginal employees may, in their confusion surrounding choice, inadvertently choose a semblance of community over none at all.

What Works

Although an aboriginal workforce can be as varied as any other, employers wishing to support a healthy work environment can prepare themselves for a number of different challenges. The loss of community, the ignorance of a corporate culture, and even the inability to choose can all be addressed by an educated view of workplace wellness. Recognizing the hazards can prepare an employer to support the growth and success of aboriginal employees.

Providing aboriginal-specific assistance through Employee Assistance Programs is essential. A look at the last 100 years of history in Canada will convince even the most doubting that trust between aboriginal and non-aboriginal people has been seriously eroded. Aboriginal employees seeking help feel much more comfortable with another aboriginal person, as there is a common link already established. It is perceived that there is no need to explain what it is to be "Indian." Non-aboriginal support workers should be careful not to present themselves as knowledgeable about aboriginal issues in order to establish a therapeutic relationship. First Nations people tend to distrust anyone who proclaims to be an "expert" on aboriginal issues. Trust will be more quickly established if the support worker acknowledges the difference between aboriginal people and mainstream society, while validating the difficulties that can arise from those differences. The diverse nature of First Nations people in this country can lead to differences between a First Nations support worker and client. The differences between those who grew up on reserve and those who did not, or those who follow traditional teachings and those who do not, can be as vast as the differences between native and non-native. Aboriginal people lost in their workplace may use race or other differences to mask the real issues. Any support worker, native or not, should be prepared for distrustful feelings from someone they are endeavouring to help.

The establishment of a community for aboriginal people in the workforce has shown remarkable success. Just as the Friendship Centre movement has provided community to off-reserve aboriginal people in urban settings, so should organizations wanting to encourage and nurture aboriginal employment look to establishing a "resource centre." The inclusion of native resources centres on campus, for example, resulted from the attempt to increase retention of students in post-secondary education. Although an actual "centre" may be unrealistic in the workplace, a bulletin board for cultural events in the area, the local aboriginal newspaper, or a yearly pow-wow listing will help connect aboriginal employees to a larger non-work-related community.

Support workers, especially peer-referral agents, need to familiarize themselves with the aboriginal community surrounding the workplace. Most large urban centres have off-reserve support services, and nearby First Nations communities can provide additional resources for employees. Peer-referral agents should visit any aboriginal organizations in the area to establish guidelines for co-operative efforts of support.

To ensure a healthy work environment for aboriginal employees, it is important to address the issue of choice. First Nations employees unfamiliar with the process of choices in the workplace may need assistance in adapting to a corporate setting. Peer-referral agents, for example, may find themselves providing career-counselling services to an aboriginal employee. Addressing the cause-and-effect of actions in the workplace, like absenteeism, may require more time and energy with an aboriginal employee. First Nations people who are unhappy with their job may need assistance in the process of changing to another job within the corporation. To identify a new position, analyze the skills or education needed for that job, and successfully apply for the job may entail skills that an aboriginal person does not currently have. Employers who can provide a service to help employees through those functions should enjoy a higher retention rate.

Employers should also be prepared to face cultural differences when enforcing corporate policy. For example, some First Nations cultures have ceremonies, attached to the death of a family member, which take place months after burial. Employees will need to be absent from work for the burial itself, then to return home for the continuation of ceremony. The very real danger of extinction of aboriginal languages and cultures can place cultural activities above workplace commitments for some First Nations employees. This may require those employees to negotiate with management for more flexible holiday time, so that they may attend traditional teachings and ceremonies.

Successful practices can be incorporated into a business setting without complete disruption of the workplace. Enaahtig Healing Lodge and Learning Centre provides residential programming to aboriginal families near Midland, Ontario. As well as incorporating traditional values into its treatment model, the Lodge also places high importance on the care of the almost completely aboriginal workforce. Cultural leave has been incorporated into the compensation package, which allows employees to attend ceremonies as they wish. Training or continuing-education programs have been expanded to recognize traditional teachings. Staff members working with elders receive the same attention as those receiving upgrading through recognized educational facilities. Processes for conflict resolution on the job include traditional elements like talking or healing circles, and staff are continually encouraged to use all available personal and community resources for self care. In fact, during non-residential programming, when client needs are less of a priority, staff are encouraged to utilize the Lodge's natural setting for their own wellness. When appropriate, staff can ride horses, or pick medicines as part of their professional functions.

Conclusion

The history, cultures, and diversity of First Nations people present challenges for workplace wellness. Understanding the presence of these challenges is the first step towards assisting aboriginal people in creating healthy workplaces for themselves. As solutions meet challenges, workplaces can become more aware of, and more sensitive to, all cultural differences in Canada's diverse society. The ability to adapt policy to need, rules to reality, and procedures to people will encourage Canada's workplace to move into a new era of health and wellness.

I can tell my children that the way to get honour
is to go to work and be good men and women.
                                    Chief Running Bird/Sequichie Hifler (1992)

References

Sequichie Hifler, J. (1992). *A Cherokee feast of days: Daily meditations*. Tulsa, OK: Council Oak Books.

Sequichie Hifler, J. (1996*). A Cherokee feast of days: Daily meditations, Volume 2.* Tulsa, OK: Council Oak Books.

22

The Next Step:
An Integrated Model of Occupational Assistance

Rick Csiernik

Introduction

We have illustrated how the workplace is a salient venue through which to address personal difficulties, as well as to assist family functioning and community health directly. Yet, what is the responsibility of counsellors to the workplace? Since the beginning of the industrial revolution in North America, an antagonistic relationship has existed between labour and management. Responsibilities of occupational counsellors have ranged from ensuring that young single women were living in virtuous Christian environments to bringing widespread use of critical incident stress debriefing to Employee Assistance Programs. These initiatives by professional counsellors supplanted self-helpers in the workplace who had become active through groups such as Alcoholics Anonymous as early as the 1940s (Brandes, 1976; McGilly, 1985; Popple, 1981; Thomlinson, 1983).

Throughout the evolution of workplace-based counselling, clinicians have retained the aura of being agents of social control (Corneil, 1984; Csiernik, 1996; Pace, 1990; Roman, 1980). However, it is hypothesized that by applying an ecological orientation to occupational assistance, and thereby attempting to create both worker and workplace wellness, one can move Employee Assistance from being a mechanism of social control to one of active social change, and a key means of enhancing workplace wellness. This process would entail integrating core practices—crisis and short-term individual and family counselling—with mutual-aid initiatives and organizational change-based theories. Taking an ecological orientation is critical given the reciprocal relationships that arise in the workplace, including both lifestyle issues and the social organization of the workplace.

Renewing Mutual Aid in the Workplace Environment

Self-help groups acted as a primary support in the development of the occupational-assistance movement (Csiernik, 1993). The industrial revolution brought with it dramatic changes in the structures of business, industry, and the state, leading to the depersonalization and dehumanization of social life, increased feelings of alienation and powerlessness, and the decline of community (Robinson & Henry, 1977). With the changing pattern of industrialization and family and social relations, new forms of mutual aid emerged to replace weakened social connections, especially in North America. Self-help groups began to respond to the depersonalization in society and became an integral aspect of co-operation between people (Katz & Bender, 1976).

As self-help evolved throughout the twentieth century from having primarily a treatment-and-normalization orientation to taking on a greater social-change direction, it has played a central role in transforming the focus of the occupational-assistance movement from tertiary to primary prevention. The growth of mutual aid/self-help outside the workplace occurred as a response to the pervasiveness of technology, the unavailability and increasing unresponsiveness of human services, the complexity and size of institutions, and the increasing dehumanizing and depersonalizing aspects of the workplace (Matzat, 1989).

Mutual aid has also been partially responsible for beginning to shift scrutiny from individual to organizational stressors that cause ill health and employee problems. Self-help has the capacity to assist and direct the evolution of occupational-assistance programs to their next plane of maturation: wellness. It has an active role in preventing occupational assistance from slipping back to being predominantly a mechanism of social control through activities such as mandatory drug testing and managed care (Ansel & Yandrick, 1993; EAPA, 1992). Self-help groups can also be one mechanism for enhancing workplace participation and democracy. They can help modify the emphasis of occupational assistance from being solely worker-centered to focusing more on problems created by the design of the workplace and the nature of the work itself. Those influenced by mutual-aid principles have the capability to act as catalysts for positive social change in the workplace, and for enhanced employee wellness; but whether that capacity will be utilized remains to be seen.

Workplace Participation

Formal employee participation in workplace decision-making is not a new concept; it has existed in a variety of forms for decades. Different organizational methods of enhancing employee participation in the workplace have emerged throughout the world. Some of the better known initiatives include Total Quality Management,[1] Quality Control Circles or simply QC Circles,[2] Theory Z of Management,[3] Quality of Working Life (QWL) enterprises,[4] and the broader industrial democracy movement.[5] While the introduction of worker participation schemes implies and requires a change in the distribution of power within a work setting, the primary, if not exclusive, theme of these exercises has been production issues. The focus of the majority of participation plans has tended to highlight more rudimentary changes, such as profit-sharing schemes, job enlargement, job rotation, and improving communication pathways, all of which involve minimal transfers of power between labourers and management. To date, participation plans that could change the nature of control over the actual decision-making processes and the work environment itself have been much less evident.

As occurred during the Gomperism era of the American labour movement, labour groups have primarily focused upon economic factors. For example, many "enlightened" European Works Councils have still concentrated their efforts on enhancing the pay packet. While this is a valid use of their energies, it has come at the cost of further enhancing the physical, psychological, social, intellectual, and spiritual health needs of the workforce. Increases in democratic initiatives do not necessarily eliminate workplace—let alone societal—inequalities. Organizational methods of worker participation are still primarily examples of representative rather than direct democratic endeavours. Individual employees in most systems make little contribution beyond their immediate work environments, with minimal attention paid to anything beyond their basic needs. Worker participation has been espoused as the next great step forward, but generally remains limited in its scope. The social and psychological elements of work have had some attention focused upon them, but the other elements of wellness still remain largely neglected. Worker participation needs to be expanded so that it encompasses an employee's total life. This is a vacuum the *Integrated Model of Occupational Assistance* begins to address.

The Integrated Model of Occupational Assistance

This model draws upon the existing practice models of occupational assistance, while placing a renewed importance on self-help. Worker participation is incorporated into an ecological framework to create an organizational plane which complements the historical emphasis upon the individual worker. The proposed model consists of two axes. The first focuses on the target. Individual wellness is balanced with organizational wellness, taking into account the needs of the range of stakeholders who exist in the immediate and extended workplace environment. The second axis is the method of intervention. It is divided into the categories of professional intervention and mutual aid/self-help. By combining both forms of assistance, four quadrants are created, allowing for a greater range of access points and prevention alternatives, and moving EAP away from being only an agent of social control (Figure 22.1).

Figure 22.1: Model Quadrants

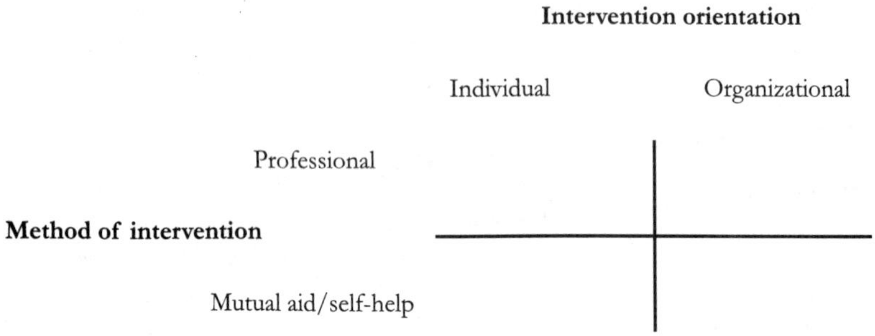

Intervention orientation

Individual   Organizational

Professional

Method of intervention

Mutual aid/self-help

i) Professional: Individual Quadrant
    The first quadrant of the *Integrated Model of Occupational Assistance* is the individual–professional intersection. It consists of activities that are, or should be, currently provided by the majority of mainstream Employee Assistance Programs and workplace health-promotion programs. These activities include ongoing health-promotion programming, together with an increased emphasis on the provision of counselling and preventative services to family members of employees and retirees. This inclusion is an acknowledgement of the fact that workplace stresses are brought home, and that home stresses brought to work by employees further intensify organizational stresses. This interrelationship manifests itself at the worksite through decreased performance and productivity. Highlighting the importance of the family within occupational assistance programming can be done in a variety of ways. Simple promotion activities, such as sending information about the program to family members, or sponsoring seminars and activities for families, are standard mechanisms. Another option is actually changing the name of this component of occupational assistance. Organizations such as

the Canadian Pacific Rail, the City of Saskatoon, MacMillan Bloedel, and the Canadian Graphic Communications Workers Alliance have already changed the name of their EAPs to "Employee and Family Assistance Programs" (EFAPs). The specific individual components of this quadrant are:

a) to provide one-to-one counselling by formally trained counselling professionals off-site or on-site, depending upon organizational needs and preferences;

b) to retain as the primary focus crisis intervention, brief counselling, and case management;

c) to promote and extend assistance to family members so that the service becomes Employee and Family Assistance Programming;

d) to provide pro-active educational seminars and workshops to the workforce by social workers and other health and counselling professionals;

e) to develop and promote activities that enhance wellness, such as voluntary health screenings conducted by occupational health staff and voluntary worksite-based fitness appraisals and programs;

f) to promote self-care activities for physical, psychological, intellectual, social, and spiritual wellness;

g) to respond to critical incidents with specially trained professional debriefers;

h) to provide 24-hour crisis intervention and consultation, accessible through a toll-free number if warranted; and,

i) to incorporate a supportive care component, so that employees absent from work for an extended period of time receive contact from the workplace to inquire if any additional non-financial assistance is required.

ii) Mutual Aid/Self-Help: Individual Quadrant

Mutual-aid initiatives have a greater potential to span the gap between wellness and traditional one-to-one counselling than do professional, individually-focused counselling services. It has been stated by various EAP stakeholder groups that peer social support could be the best potential bridge between health promotion, prevention programming, and Employee Assistance Programming (Csiernik, 1995).

While the issue of confidentiality will always arise when discussing EAPs, this has not been a hindrance to many existing programs with very active self-help components.[6] Self-help can be introduced through a variety of means. If there is uncertainty about how a mutual-aid initiative will be received by a workforce, it would be judicious to begin initially with a physical health-related or psycho-educational focused group. Treatment-orientated groups could be considered if a specific request occurs from members of the workforce, or, of course, if a group arises spontaneously. For many organizations, on-site mutual-aid/self-help groups will be much easier to support if they are focused upon wellness themes or upon issues of daily living such as child care or the demands of aging parents. Components of this quadrant are:

a) the use of peers, union counsellors, referral agents, peer resource teams, and/or peer advisors to give employees access to appropriate forms of assistance and to provide on-going social support;

b) the use of community-based self-help groups as an adjunct to individual assistance and to further enhance social support;

c) the development of on-site self-help groups that deal with traditional problem areas and with wellness-related topics if the employee population is large enough or if distinct work-site-specific problems arise and requests emerge; and,

d) a timely response to any critical incident situation with trained peer debriefers who understand the culture of the organization and the nature of the routine stresses, as well as the potential range of stress reactions produced by a critical incident.

iii) Professional: Organizational Quadrant

The third quadrant moves occupational counselling into a new realm. It offers increased possibilities for organization-wide primary prevention and more pro-active initiatives, including counsellors acting as mediators between individuals and between work units in an alternative dispute resolution process. The activities within this quadrant recognize that workplace health does not simply relate to employees' engaging in healthy behaviours but also includes making the work environment healthier. This would enhance the probability that both individual risk factors and broader environmental and structural issues would be integrated into program undertakings.

This quadrant also introduces the idea that occupational assistance can, and should, enter into the broader context of policy change and advocacy beyond the workplace. There is a place for workplace wellness to be discussed and debated at societal and political levels. While the immediate impact of this aspect of the model may be minimal, in the long term it could be the most important dimension in creating not only well workplaces but also healthier communities. Advocacy efforts may come from researchers or professional associations as well as from groups with vested interests in the workplace. Examples of these are Chambers of Commerce, the Canadian Labour Congress, and government-mandated health and safety associations such as the Industrial Accident Prevention Association (IAPA), along with professional associations such as the Canadian Association of Social Workers. Goals of the third quadrant are:

a)   to provide ongoing work-site-wide health promotion, safety, and critical-incident awareness and related wellness education programs;

b)   to provide consultation and training for ongoing organizational intervention, development, and change, including team-building initiatives;

c)   to enhance the health of work units through the provision of technical assistance, including mediation or conflict-resolution services on both individual and organizational issues; and,

d)   to collaborate with individuals and groups external to the work-site in advocating for policy initiatives to increase the wellness and productivity of the workforce, to enhance the healthy functioning of workplaces, and to increase the profile of occupational assistance.

iv)   Mutual Aid/Self-Help: Organizational Quadrant

The fourth segment of the model is the organizational mutual-aid/self-help dimension. Programming arising from this quadrant reflects the needs of labour and management to work conjointly to define, identify, and diagnose organizationally created problems. The two groups need to work together to find and implement solutions that can counter organizationally produced reductions in both productivity and wellness. There are two primary options for these types of support groups: either broad organization-wide groups open to all employees, or groups organized along departmental or work-unit lines. The organizational culture will be the predominant factor in determining whether either or both types of groups emerge. Training and education about these teams (which are rarely done prior to implementation), how to use them, and their strengths and limitations would be essential steps in properly developing the goals identified in this quadrant. Beginning the process by providing training would be far preferable to simply telling employees that they were being placed in teams, and expecting them to know how to function in this new manner, not to mention expecting them to function more efficiently. The education process that precedes this dimension could be conducted by peers or by professionals internal or external to the workplace (discussed above in the professional/ organizational quadrant). The three goals of this quadrant are:

a) to engage in team-building exercises and activities in order to acquaint the workforce with expectations, rights, and responsibilities of being a team or group member;

b) to develop mutual-aid group(s), open to all employees, which examine stressors both internal and external to the workplace affecting individual and group wellness;

c) to develop work-unit support groups to decrease work-related stress and to act as problem-solving and/or peer social-support groups.

Conclusion

The *Integrated Model of Occupational Assistance* is premised upon the idea that to achieve wellness—physical, psychological, social, intellectual, and spiritual—the workplace needs to address both production and personal issues. The various ideas all hinge—to varying degrees—on the belief that participatory democracy is a valuable commodity toward which all workplaces should be evolving. Locke, Schweiger, and Latham (1984) claimed that participation is not simply an ethical imperative, but also a core managerial technique which is appropriate in any situation. However, in occupational programming, participation should not only be deemed ethically correct, but also should become a professional mandate. Employee Assistance counselling professionals and peer supports need to place greater value on self-determination and regard it as one of the core foundations for all human interaction and development, not only outside the workplace but within it as well.

The delivery of the *Integrated Model of Occupational Assistance* is intended to be flexible, with a range of implementation options. An organization may begin by developing a physical health promotion component before adding other health promotion or treatment elements. An organization that has a traditional Employee Assistance Program in place could easily incorporate the mutual-aid/self-help dimension. These options allow for mutual aid/ self-help or organization intervention dimensions to be added to mature occupational assistance programs or to be a foundation for new programming.

Implementation will of course be dependent upon the nature of the workplace and workforce. Presentation of the model to workplaces may be sufficiently vague and generic to allow each organization to take ownership of the program's evolution and adapt the different elements to its own needs.

The intent of this second-generation model of occupational assistance is to move away from the notion of intervention as social control. Its goal is not to isolate but rather to integrate physical, social, and organizational aspects of the workplace with behavioural and lifestyle aspects of work. It is structured in a manner that, when fully implemented, should improve the overall functioning of the workplace and the health of employees and their families. Counsellors involved in occupational assistance, because of their knowledge, skills, entry points, and positioning in organizations, have the opportunity to improve the quality of life for workers by becoming active change agents and encouraging participatory democratic action. However, occupational assistance is but a small sub-system of any organization. Programs and their champions cannot control all acts of employers, and there are inherent limits on what can be realistically accomplished. Thus, to change workplace wellness also requires changes in our cultural norms, public and social policy, labour legislation, and existing institutions. This is a noble goal for all involved in this enterprise.

Endnotes
1. Deming 1938; 1950; Ishikawa, 1985; Juran and Gryna, Jr., 1970.
2. Crocker, Chiu, & Charney, 1984; Dewar, 1980.
3. Ouchi, 1981.
4. Ferman, 1985; Giordano, 1992; Ingle & Ingle, 1983; Kolodny & van Beinum, 1983.
5. Davies, 1979; Emery & Thorsrud, 1969; Obradovic & Dunn, 1978; Prasnikar, 1991.
6. Bisgona, 1992; Csiernik, 2002; Eisman, 1991; Grant, 1992; Windsor, 1988.

References

Ansel, D. & Yandrick, R. (1993). Building and integrated EAP-managed behavioural health care program: Tying up loose ends. *EAPA Exchange* 23(3), 33–35.

Bisogna, G. (1992). Surviving recession. *EAP Digest* 12(3), 12, 40–41.

Brandes, S. (1976). *American welfare capitalism, 1880–1940*. Chicago: University of Chicago Press.

Corneil, W. (1984). History, philosophy and objectives of an employee recovery program. In W. Albert, B. Boyle, & C. Ponee (eds.), *EAP Orientation: Volume II—Important Concepts*. Toronto: Addiction Research Foundation.

Crocker, O., Chiu, J., Sik L., & Charney, C. (1984). *Quality circles: A guide to participation and productivity.* Toronto: Methuen.

Csiernik, R. (1993). The role of mutual aid/self-help in North American occupational assistance: Past, present and future. *Employee Assistance Quarterly* 9(2), 21–45.

Csiernik, R. (1995). An integrated model of occupational assistance. Unpublished dissertation, University of Toronto.

Csiernik, R. (1996). Occupational social work: From social control to social assistance? *The Social Worker* 64(3), 67–74.

Csiernik, R. (2002). An overview of Employee and Family Assistance Programming in Canada. *Employee Assistance Quarterly* 18(1), 17–33.

Davies, R. (1979). Industrial democracy in international perspective. In G. Sanderson & F. Stapenhurst (eds.), *Industrial democracy today.* Toronto: McGraw-Hill Ryerson.

Deming, W. E. (1938). *Statistical adjustment of data.* New York: Dover.

Deming, W. E. (1950). *Some theory of sampling.* New York: John Wiley and Sons.

Dewar, D. (1980). *The quality circle guide to participation management.* Englewood Cliffs: Prentice-Hall.

EAPA. (1992). Outcome studies. *EAPA Exchange* 22(10), 48–49.

Eisman, C. (1991) Is corporate America about to embrace self-help groups? *Self-Helper* 6(2), 1–5.

Emery, F.E. & Thorsrud, E. (1969). *Form and content in industrial democracy.* London: Tavistock.

Ferman, L. (1985). Quality of work–life programs and EAPs: The reorganization of the workplace. In S. Klarreich, J. Francek, and C. Moore (eds.), *The human resource management handbook.* Toronto: Praeger Press.

Giordano, L. (1992). *Beyond Taylorism: Computerization and the new industrial relations.* New York: St. Martin's Press.

Grant, G. (1992). Workplace peer power. *EAPA Exchange* 22(8), 22–25.

Ingle, S. & Ingle, N. (1983). *Quality circles in service industries.* Englewood Cliffs: Prentice-Hall.

Ishikawa, K. (1985). *What is total quality control? The Japanese way.* Englewood Cliffs: Prentice-Hall.

Juran, J.M. & Gryna, Frank, Jr. (1970). *Quality planning and analysis.* Toronto: McGraw-Hill.

Katz, A. & Bender, E. (1976). *The strength in us.* New York: New Viewpoints.

Kerans, P., Dorver, G., & Williams, D. (1988). *Welfare and worker participation.* New York: St. Martin's Press.

Kolodny, H. & van Beinum, H. (1983). *The quality of working life and the 1980s.* New York: Praeger.

Locke, E., Schweiger, D., & Latham, G. (1984). Participation in decision making: When should it be used? *Organizational Dynamics* 14(3), 65–79.

Matzat, J. (1989). Some remarks on West Germany's health and welfare system and the position of self-help. In S. Humble & J. Unell (eds.), *Self-help in health and social welfare*. New York: Routledge.

McGilly, F. (1985). American historical antecedents to industrial social work. *Social work papers of the School of Social Work, University of Southern California* 19, 1–13.

Obradovic, J. & Dunn, W. (1978). *Worker's self-management and organizational power in Yugoslavia*. Pittsburgh: University of Pittsburgh.

Ouchi, W. (1981). *Theory Z*. New York: Avon.

Pace, E. (1990). Peer Employee Assistance Programs for nurses. *Perspectives on addictions nursing* 1(4), 3–7.

Popple, P. (1981). Social work practice in business and industry, 1875–1930. *Social Service Review* 55, 257–269.

Prasnikar, J. (1991). *Workers' participation and self-management in developing countries*. San Francisco: Westview Press.

Robin, M. (1968). *Radical politics and Canadian labour*. Kingston: Industrial Relations Centre.

Robinson, D. & Henry, S. (1977). *Self-help and health*. Bungay: Chaucer Press.

Roman, P. (1980). Medicalization and social control in the workplace: prospects for the 1980s. *Journal of Applied Behavioural Science* 16(3), 407–422.

Stephens, E. (1980). *The politics of workers' participation*. Toronto: Academic Press.

Thomlison, R. (1983). Industrial social work: Perspectives and Issues. In R. Thomlinson (ed.), *Perspectives on industrial social work*. Toronto: Family Service Canada.

Windsor, R., Lowe, J., & Bartlett, E. (1988). The effectiveness of a worksite self-help smoking cessation program: A randomized trial. *Journal of Behavioural Medicine* 11(4), 407–421.

List of Contributing Authors

Rick Csiernik

Rick is Professor of Social Work and Coordinator of Graduate Studies at King's University College at the University of Western Ontario. He earned both BSc and BSW degrees at McMaster University; a MSW and PhD in Social Work from the University of Toronto, where he specialized in Employee Assistance Studies; and a Graduate Diploma in Social Administration from Wilfrid Laurier University. Former coordinator of the McMaster University EAP Studies program and the first president of the Canadian Employee Assistance Program Association, Rick has presented and consulted on EAP issues across Canada and has authored over 100 publications, including co-editing *Responding to the Oppression of Addiction: Canadian Social Work Perspectives* with Dr. William S. Rowe (also published by Canadian Scholars' Press). The remainder of his time is spent coaching, managing, and watching his sons' (Alexander and Benjamin) hockey, baseball, and basketball teams.

David W. Adams

David, BScN, MSW, RSW, CDE, CT, is currently a private therapist, facilitator, and mediation consultant. He is Professor Emeritus, Department of Psychiatry and Behavioural Neurosciences, Faculty of Health Sciences, McMaster University; and was formerly Executive Director of the Greater Hamilton Employee Assistance Consortium and Hurst Place: The Employee Assistance Program. Prior to this David was the founding Director of Social Work Services and Co-Director Psychosocial Program, McMaster University Medical Centre; and Chair, Patient Relations Council, Chedoke–McMaster Hospitals. He is particularly interested in the mediation of workplace and family conflicts, management of the impact of harassment and violence, provision of effective rehabilitation in trauma and stress-induced illnesses, and the treatment of the complications of loss and grief in individuals and families. Recent areas of study include the pivotal role of spirituality in life challenges and professional education, the value of mediation versus litigation, and the parameters of suffering and healing. During his career, David has been internationally recognized as a lecturer, workshop facilitator, and author. He served for many years as Professional Advisor to the Candlelighters Childhood Cancer Foundation Canada, was elected Chair of the International Work Group on Death, Dying and Bereavement (IWG), and was appointed to the Ontario Council of Health, the senior policy advisory body to the Ontario Minister of Health.

Susan Alexander

Susan received her BSW from King's University College at the University of Western Ontario, and her MSW from the University of Toronto. She is currently a social worker within the London Health Sciences Centre, engaged in emergency/trauma care within the paediatric emergency service. Her work entails the psychosocial treatment of children and families in crisis from a host of issues, including sudden death, physical and sexual abuse, acute mental breakdown, acute critical illness, and acute stress intervention. Susan also has a private practice working with individuals and families, and is a part-time faculty member in the School of Social Work at King's University College at the University of Western Ontario, London, Ontario.

Brenda Atkinson

Brenda has an MSW and is a registered social worker and registered marital and family therapist. She is a supervisor at WestBridge Associates Employee Assistance Service, an external provider of EAP services in London, Ontario.

Kelly Brownbill

Kelly, whose spirit name "Wabunnoongakekwe" means "Woman Who Comes From the East," has worked for the largest single-site employer of First Nation people in Canada for the past ten years. Her primary responsibilities are to provide peer support services to the aboriginal employees and First Nation Awareness training programs to all staff. A proud member of the Mi'kmaq Nation and the Marten Clan, Kelly also works with a number of aboriginal initiatives on a volunteer basis to promote wellness for her people. She honours the wisdom and vision of her elders, both here and in the spirit realm, and acknowledges their guidance.

Rick Cooper

Rick is the past Director of WestBridge Associates Employee Assistance Service, an external provider of EAP services in London, Ontario. He has an MSW and is a registered social worker.

Jan Devereux

Jan, a registered social worker, has her MSW and is Team Leader Manager, Medical Services, St. Joseph's Health Centre, London, Ontario, and also serves as a member of the Employee Counselling Service Advisory Committee.

Sandra Ferreira

Sandy received her Bachelor of Social Work from King's University College in London, Ontario. She has worked as a research assistant for Professor Dermot Hurley of King's University College and is currently a case worker with Big Brothers in London, Ontario.

Tony Fasulo

Tony is both a founder and managing partner of Acclaim Ability Management Inc., a national disability-management company. He is a graduate of the National Institute of Disability Management and Research (NIDMAR) certification program, a Registered Rehabilitation Professional, a seasoned Vocational Evaluator, and has his designation as an Associate in Life Health Claims (International Claims Association). Tony has garnered professional experience as Director of Psychosocial Rehabilitation Services for the Canadian Mental Health Association, as well through his management position in the disability-management industry for over a decade.

Louise Hartley

Louise is a registered psychologist who received her doctorate in clinical psychology from York University. Her 28 years of experience in many different settings—education, children's mental health, hospitals, and business—have given her a broad base of knowledge in helping people cope with numerous types of problems. She has developed expertise in the field of organizational development that includes both individual and team interventions designed to build healthy work environments. Louise is Vice President Clinical Services at Family Services Employee Assistance Programs (FSEAP) in Toronto, providing executive coaching services to help companies retain and develop their high-potential employees. She is a frequent speaker at conferences on the topics of organizational health and depression in the workplace. Louise is President of the Employee Assistance Society of North America (EASNA) and is also President of the Employee Assistance Program Association of Toronto.

Marilyn A. Herie

Marilyn has been a therapist and project leader at the Centre for Addiction and Mental Health (CAMH) since 1992, and is currently an Education Specialist in the Education and Publishing Department. She is also an Adjunct Professor at the Faculty of Social Work, University of Toronto, and coordinates the Collaborative Program in Addiction Studies at the Faculty of Social Work. Her focus at CAMH has been on the development and dissemination of research-based practice protocols, including Structured Relapse Prevention (1996), Guided Self-Change for EAPs (1996), the Back on Track Mandatory Remedial Measures Program (2000), as well as, more recently, the development and evaluation of online courses. In addition, Marilyn is a clinical trainer and therapist specializing in the group and individual treatment of adults with alcohol/drug problems. Marilyn has facilitated hundreds of workshops and presented at academic conferences throughout Canada and in other countries. She has co-authored books, book chapters, and articles in scholarly journals on brief treatment, alcohol dependence, relapse prevention, dissemination research, and online learning. Marilyn also teaches an online course on addiction treatment in the Faculty of Social Work, University of Toronto. She received her doctorate in social work at the University of Toronto, where she conducted research on web-based continuing education for therapists and health-care practitioners.

Dermott Hurley

Dermott is an Assistant Professor of Social Work at King's University College at the University of Western Ontario, London, Ontario. He has 25 years' experience working with children, adolescents, and families in various crisis situations; he specializes in trauma and bereavement counselling, and currently consults to the Psychiatric Trauma Team at London Health Sciences Centre. He is also affiliated with the Department of Psychiatry at the University of Western Ontario.

Penny Lawson

Penny, an International Certified Alcohol and Drug Counsellor, is Manager, Family Services and Special Programs, for Bellwood Health

Services and is a charter member of the Bellwood Staff, having worked in the field of addiction since 1982. In addition to her managerial duties, Penny is responsible for Bellwood's Relapse Prevention Program, Problem Gambling Program, Family Program, CSD/PTSD Program, Outpatient Counselling, Intervention Services, Sexual Addiction Program, and Training Services. She also co-ordinates special programs such as wellness and stress. Penny has an extensive educational background in addiction, and is an experienced presenter and trainer of professionals who are to expand their understanding of chemical dependency.

Within Canada she has presented at the McMaster Institute on Addiction Studies, the Justice Department of the Northwest Territories, the Department of National Defense, Pauktuutit, the Inuit Women's Institute, Centennial College, and many community organizations and conferences. Internationally she has made presentations in the United States, Trinidad and Tobago, and Antigua. In addition to her work with Bellwood, Penny maintains an active private practice in Toronto.

Frank MacAuley

Frank hails from Prince Edward Island, where he has spent his professional social work career since receiving his MSW from Carleton University in 1973. Frank has studied the effect of stress on the body and has received advanced Certificates in Mind–Body Medicine from Harvard University Medical School and the Mindfulness-Based Stress Reduction Program at the Omega Institute, New York. Since 1989 Frank has been Clinical Manager of the Internal EAP for public sector employees within the government of Prince Edward Island. He also has a private practice, having recently formed Atlantic Employee Assistance Providers with two colleagues. Nationally, Frank has been active in the Canadian EAP Association, developing advanced practice guidelines and standards for practitioners.

Scott Macdonald

Scott is Associate Professor in Health Information Science at the University of Victoria, and Assistant Director of the Centre for Addictions Research in Victoria, British Columbia. His educational background includes degrees in Psychology (BSc), Criminology (MA), and Epidemiology (PhD). Scott has written extensively on drug testing in the workplace, and has been an expert witness in several cases related to substance abuse in the workplace. His workplace research includes empirical studies on occupational risk factors for alcohol and drug problems, evaluations of the impact of Employee Assistance Programs on employee health and productivity, and the impact of drug testing on workplace injuries. He is currently conducting a large-scale survey of Canadian workplaces to assess the nature and extent of EAPs, health promotion, and drug testing programs.

Sara Martel

Sara received her MA from York University/Ryerson University's Communication and Culture Joint Program in Toronto, Ontario. She also holds a Combined Honours BA in English Literature and Media Information & Technoculture from the University of Western Ontario in London, Ontario. Sara is currently responsible for national communications at Acclaim Ability Management Inc. Much of the research, conference and seminar presentations, industry publication articles, and other literature Sara has produced relates to prevalent disability-management issues such as psychosocial health and integrated workplace wellness.

Claire Pain

Claire received her Diploma of Physiotherapy from Middlesex Hospital in London, England, her BSc in Physiotherapy from the University of Toronto, and then completed her MSc and her MD at McMaster University in Hamilton, Ontario. She served her psychiatric residency at the University of Ottawa and previously served as general duty medical officer at the National Defense Headquarters and National Defense Medical Center in Ottawa, Ontario. Claire is currently staff psychiatrist and clinical director of the psychological trauma and assessment clinic at Mount Sinai Hospital in Toronto, Ontario, and is also an assistant professor at the University of Toronto, Department of Psychiatry.

Hilda Sabadash

Hilda is the Program Coordinator of Bereaved Families of Ontario–Ottawa Region (BFO-OR). Since 1998, she has coordinated support groups with trained volunteer facilitators and offers public education sessions to schools, corporations and institutions. BFO–OR's mandate is to offer peer support to anyone after the death of a loved one. Following personal loss, Hilda took the BFO–OR training to be a facilitator and for five years co-facilitated groups for loss of a spouse. Hilda is a former registered nurse, has a Palliative Care Certificate, Pastoral Care Certificate, and is a lay preacher in the Ottawa area with the United Church of Canada.

Debbie Samson

Debbie, a Certified Employee Assistance Professional, has been coordinator of the Employee Assistance Program at the Iron Ore Company of Canada in Labrador, Canada since its inception in 1990. Debbie is a graduate of the

Addiction Studies Program and the Employee Assistance Studies Program at McMaster University, Hamilton, Ontario. Debbie has lived in the mining town of Labrador City, Newfoundland with her husband, Bill, and two children, Lisa and William, for over 25 years. She may be contacted at the Employee Assistance Program, Iron Ore Company of Canada, PO Box 1000, Labrador City, Newfoundland, A2V 2L8, samsond@ironore.ca.

Wayne Skinner

Wayne is Deputy Clinical Director in the Addictions Program at the Centre for Addiction and Mental Health in Toronto. He is also an Assistant Professor in the Department of Psychiatry at the University of Toronto, and an adjunct senior lecturer in its Faculty of Social Work; in addition, he teaches part-time in the School of Social Work at York University, Toronto. As Head of Outpatient Services at the Addiction Research Foundation in the 1980s, Wayne co-developed one of the first manualized, evidence-based brief outpatient treatment programs in Canada. His interest in Brief Treatment has continued since that time, sharpened by a range of clinical experience; this includes EAP counselling and private practice, as well as working in an institutional setting in a large metropolitan area.

His clinical research interests include telecounselling, mutual aid for people with addictions, supporting families affected by mental health and addiction problems, and the treatment of anger problems. He has presented at workshops nationally and internationally, and is currently editing a book on the treatment of concurrent disorders.

Mary Young

Mary, a certified social worker, was the coordinator of the internal component of St. Joseph's Employee Counselling Service (London, Ontario) prior to her retirement.

Copyright Acknowledgments